FRACTAL PHYSIOLOGY
AND
CHAOS IN MEDICINE

Studies of Nonlinear Phenomena in Life Science — Vol. 1

FRACTAL PHYSIOLOGY
AND
CHAOS IN MEDICINE

Bruce J. West
Department of Physics
University of North Texas
USA

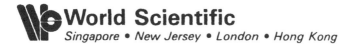
World Scientific
Singapore • New Jersey • London • Hong Kong

Published by

World Scientific Publishing Co. Pte. Ltd.

P O Box 128, Farrer Road, Singapore 912805

USA office: Suite 1B, 1060 Main Street, River Edge, NJ 07661

UK office: 57 Shelton Street, Covent Garden, London WC2H 9HE

British Library Cataloguing-in-Publication Data
A catalogue record for this book is available from the British Library.

First published 1990
Reprinted 1998, 2000

FRACTAL PHYSIOLOGY AND CHAOS IN MEDICINE

ISBN 981-02-0127-3
ISBN 981-02-0128-1 (pbk)

Printed in Singapore.

This book is dedicated to my wife Sharon
for her love and understanding.

Preface for Second Printing

I am gratified that this small book is going into a second printing. If time had allowed I might have updated the examples given in the last chapter and winnowed out some of the more speculative comments sprinkled throughout. However, much that was tentative and speculative ten years ago, has since become well documented, if not universally accepted. So if I had started down the road of revision I could easily have written an entirely new book. Upon rereading the text I decided that it accomplished its original purpose rather well, that being, to communicate to a broad audience the recent advances in modeling that have had, and are continuing to have, a significant influence on physiology and medicine. So I decided to leave well enough alone.

Bruce J. West
Research Triangle Park, NC
January 1, 2000

Preface

This book is concerned with the application of *fractals* and *chaos* (as well as other concepts from nonlinear dynamics systems theory) to biomedical phenomena. In particular, I have used biomedical data sets and modern mathematical concepts to argue against the outdated notion of homeostasis. It seems to me that health is at least a homeodynamic process with multiple steady states – each being capable of survival. This idea was developed in collaboration with my friend and colleague A. Goldberger during long discussions in which we attempted to learn each other's disciplines. This book is not restricted to our own research, however, but draws from the research of a large number of investigators. Herein we seek breadth rather than depth in order to communicate some of the excitement being experienced by scientists making applications of these concepts in the life sciences.

I have tried in most cases to motivate a new mathematical concept using a biomedical data set and have avoided discussing mathematics for its own sake. Herein the phenomena to be explained take precedence over the mathematics and therefore one will not find any proofs, but some attempt has been made to provide reference as to where such proofs can be found.

I wish to thank all those who have provided help and inspiration over the years, in particular L. Glass, A. Goldberger, A. Mandell and M. Shlesinger; with special thanks to A. Babloyantz for a critical reading of an early version of the manuscript. I also wish to thank Ms. Rosalie Rocher for her expert word processing of the manuscript and W. Deering for making the time to complete this work available to me.

Bruce J. West
Denton, Texas
July 4, 1990

Table of Contents

1. INTRODUCTION

The driver dozing behind the wheel of a car speeding along the highway, the momentary lapse in concentration of the airtraffic controller, or the continuous activity of an airplane pilot could all benefit from a diagnostic tuned to the activity of the brain associated with wakeful attentiveness. As systems become more complex and operators are required to handle ever-increasing amounts of data and rapidly make decisions, the need for such a diagnostic becomes more and more clear. The development of new techniques to assess the state of the operator in real time may have recently become available, so that in the near future the capability may exist for alerting the operator, or someone in the command structure, to the possibility of impending performance breakdown. This is an example of how new ideas for understanding dynamics systems may be used in biomedical/social systems.

We are now in the position where clinicians with their stethoscopes poised over the healthy heart, radiologists tracking the flow of blood and bile, and physiologists probing the nervous system are all, for the most part unknowingly, exploring the frontiers of chaos and fractals. These related topics are central concepts in the new discipline of *nonlinear dynamics* developed in physics and mathematics. Perhaps the most compelling applications of these concepts are not in the physical sciences but rather in physiology and medicine where fractals and chaos may radically change long-held views about order and variability in health and disease. What we attempt to document here is that a healthy physiological system has a certain amount of intrinsic variability, and a transition to a more ordered or less complicated state may be indicative of disease. For example, the healthy variability in the normal mammalian heart is lost when the cardiac activity undergoes ventricular fibrillation, a state in which the normal spectrum of the cardiac pulse narrows.

Goldberger, Rigney and West (1990) pointed out previously that the conventional wisdom in medicine holds disease and aging to arise from stress on an otherwise orderly and machine-like system. It is believed that this stress decreases order by provoking erratic responses or by upsetting the body's normal periodic rhythms. Investigators have, over the past five years or so, discovered that the heart and other physiological systems may behave most erratically when they are young and healthy. Counterintuitively, increasingly regular behavior sometimes accompanies aging and disease. Thus, irregularity and unpredictability are important features of health.

The above authors go on to point out that for at least five decades physicians have interpreted the normal operation of physiological systems to be the reduction in variability and maintenance of a constant internal function: the principle of homeostasis. According to this theory, developed by Walter B. Cannon of the Harvard Medical School, any physiological variable should return to its "normal" steady-state operation after it has been perturbed. In their article the authors argue, as we do here, that the notion of homeostasis is atavistic and one might more reasonably associate a principle of homeodynamics with the present day understanding of biomedical processes. Such a principle would require the existence of multiple metastable states for any physiological variable rather than a single steady state. The erratic behavior of healthy physiological systems would not be interpreted as transient perturbations of the systems to a fluctuating environment, but rather the normal "chaotic" behavior would be associated with a new paradigm of health. The articulation of such a principle is probably premature, but the mounting evidence appears to support its existence.

We review herein such esoteric concepts as strange attractors, the generators of chaos in many situations, and argue that far from being unusual, they may be dynamical maps of healthy fluctuations in the heart, brain and other organs observed under most ordinary circumstances. Broad spectra of time series representing the dynamic behavior of a biological system appear to be markers of physiological information, not "noise." Thus rather than neglecting such irregular behavior we must learn how to extract the information contained therein.

The activity of cardiac pulses and brain waves are quite similar to a wide variety of other natural phenomena that exhibit irregular and apparently unpredictable or random behavior. Examples that immediately come to mind are the changes in the weather over a few days time, the height of the next wave breaking on the beach as you sit in the hot sun, shivering from a cold wind blowing down your back, and the infuriating intermittency in the time intervals between the drips from the bathroom faucet just after you crawl into bed at night. In some cases such as the weather, the phenomenon appears to be always random, but in other cases such as the dripping faucet, sometimes the dripping is periodic and other times each drip appears to be independent of the preceding one, thereby forming a irregular sequence (Shaw, 1981). The formal property that all these phenomena share is nonlinearity, so that our initial investigation focuses on how non-linear models may differ from linear ones. In particular we examine how simple non-linearities can generate aperiodic processes, and consequently apparently random phenomena in a brainwave context (Basar, 1985) in a cardiac environment (Goldberger and West, 1987) and in a broad range of other biomedical situations.

1.1 What is Linearity?

Nonlinearity is one of those strange concepts that is defined by what it is not. As more than one physicist has put it: "It is like having a zoo of non-elephants." Thus we need to identify clearly the properties of linearity in order to specify which property a particular nonlinear process does not have. Consider, for example, a complicated system that consists of a number of factors. One property of linearity is that the response of the action of each separate factor is proportional to its value. This is the *property of proportionality*. Consider the response of a well-oiled swing to being pushed. The height attained by the swing is directly proportional to how hard it is pushed, assuming that it does not rotate about the support bar or the chains do not become slack as the swing returns etc. Each of these *extraordinary* effects destroys the linearity of the swing. Therefore we say the swing (or pendulum to give a more rigid example) is linear for gentle pushes but becomes increasingly nonlinear as the applied force is increased.

A second property of linearity is that the total response of the system to an action is equal to the sum of the results of the values of the separate factors. This is the *property of independence*; see eq. Faddeev (1964). Pushing a stalled automobile on level ground exemplifies this effect. The more individuals one can convince to impel the vehicle, the greater is its subsequent speed prior to releasing the clutch.

As an example of linearity we choose systems theory, since this discipline has been used for a number of years in the analysis of biomedical time series including brain wave data and in interpreting the response of this activity to external stimulations (Basar, 1976). In the standard theory one asserts that a process (or system) is linear if the output of an operation is directly proportional to the input. The proportionality constant is a measure of the sensitivity of the system to the input. Formally the response, R, of a physical system is linear when it is directly proportional to the applied force F. This relation can be expressed algebraically by the relation $R = \alpha F + \beta$, where α and β are constants. If there is no response in the absence of the applied force, then $\beta = 0$. This is the algebraic expression of the swing response discussed above. In a linear system if two distinct forces F_1 and F_2 are applied, the net response would be $R = \alpha_1 F_1 + \alpha_2 F_2$, where α_1 and α_2 are independent constants. If there are N independent applied forces denoted by the vector $\mathbf{F} = (F_1, F_2, \ldots, F_N)$ then the response of the system is linear if there is a vector $\alpha = (\alpha_1, \alpha_2, \ldots, \alpha_N)$ of independent constant components such that $R = \alpha \cdot \mathbf{F} = \sum_{j=1}^{N} \alpha_j F_j$. In this last equation, we see that the total response of the system, here a scalar, is a sum of the independent applied forces F_j each weighted by its own sensitivity coefficient α_j. These ideas carry over to more general systems where $\mathbf{F}$ is a generalized time dependent force vector and R is the generalized response.

As discussed by Lavrentév and Nikol'skii (1964) one of the most fruitful and brilliant ideas of the second half of the 1600's was the idea that the concept of a function and the geometric representation of a line are related. Geometrically the notion of a linear relation between two quantities implies that if a graph is constructed with the ordinate denoting the values of one variable and the abscissa denoting the values of the other variables then the relation in question appears as a straight line. In systems of more than two variables, a linear relation defines a higher order "flat" surface. For example, three variables can be realized as a three dimensional coordinate space, and the linear relation defines a plane in this space. One often sees this notion employed in the analysis of data by first transforming one or more of the variables to a form in which the data is anticipated to lie on a straight line. Thus one often searches for a representation in which linear ideas may be valid since the analysis of linear systems is completely understood, whereas that for nonlinear systems of various kinds is still relatively primitive (West, 1983).

The two notions of linearity that we have expressed here, algebraic and geometric, although equivalent, have quite different implications. The latter use of the idea is a static graph of a function expressed as the geometrical locus of the points where coordinates satisfy a linear relationship. The former expression in our examples has to do with the response of a system to an applied force which implies that the system is dynamic, i.e., the physical observables change over time even though the force-response relation may be independent of time. This change of the observable in time is referred to as the evolution of the system and for only the simplest systems is the relation between the dependent and independent variables a linear one. We will have ample opportunity to explore the distinction between the above static and dynamic notions of linearity. It should be mentioned that if the axes for the graphical display exhaust the independent variables that describe the system, then the two interpretations dovetail.

The state of a given system is defined by a point in this latter graph, often called either the state space or phase space of the system. The state of a system is a complete specification of all the independent variables needed to describe the system at a given instant of time. In the swing example, specifying the height of the swing or equivalently its angular position, completely determines the instantaneous state of the swing. The swing after all is one-dimensional. As time moves on the point traces out a curve, called an orbit or trajectory, that describes the history of the system's evolution. Each point in phase space is a state of the system. Thus an orbit gives the sequence of states occupied by the system through time, but does not indicate how long the system occupies a particular state. Such details are discussed subsequently. This geometrical representation of dynamics is one of the most useful tools in dynamic systems theory for analyzing the time-dependent properties of nonlinear systems. By nonlinear we now know that we mean the output of the system is not proportional to the input. One implication of this is the following: If the system is linear, then two trajectories initiated at nearby points in phase space would evolve in close proximity, so that at any point in future time the two trajectories (and therefore the states of the system they represent) would also be near one another. If the system is nonlinear then two such trajectories could diverge from one another and at subsequent times (exactly how long will be discussed subsequently) the two trajectories would be arbitrarily far apart, i.e., the distance between the orbits does not evolve in a proportionate way. Of course this need not necessarily happen in a nonlinear system; it is a question of stability.

The accepted criteria for understanding a given phenomena varies as one changes from discipline to discipline since different disciplines are at different levels of scientific maturity. In the early developmental stage of a discipline one is often satisfied with characterizing a phenomenon be means of a detailed verbal description. This stage of development reaches maturity when general concepts are introduced which tie together observations by means of one or few basic principles, e.g., Darwin (1859) did this with evolution through the introduction of: (1) the principle of universal evolution, (2) the law of natural selection, and (3) the law of survival of the fittest. Freud (1895) did this with human behavior through the introduction of concepts such as conversion hysteria and neuroses. These investigators postulated causal relations using repeated observations of the gross properties of the systems they examined. As observational techniques became more refined additional detailed structures associated with these gross properties were uncovered. In the examples cited the genetic structure of the DNA molecule has for some replaced Darwin's notion of "survival of the fittest" and causal relations for social behavior are now sought at the level of biochemistry (see e.g. Dawkins, 1976). The schism between Freud's vision of a grand psychoanalytic theory and micro-biology is no less great. The criteria for understanding the later stages of development are quite different from those in the first stage. At these "deeper" levels the underlying principles must be universal and tied to the disciplines of mathematics, physics, and chemistry. This is no less true for medicine as we pass from the clinical diagnosis of a ailment to its laboratory cure. Thus concepts such as energy and entropy appear in the discussion of microbiological processes and are used to guide the progress of research in these areas.

The mathematical models that have historically developed throughout natural philosophy have followed the paradigms of physics and chemistry. Not just in the search for basic postulates that will be universally applicable and from which one can draw deductions, but more restrictively at the operational level the techniques that have been adopted, with few exceptions, have been *linear*. One example of this, the implications of which will prove to be quite important in physiology, has to do with the ability to isolate and measure, i.e., to operationally define, a variable. In natural philosophy this operational definition of a variable becomes intertwined with the concept of linearity and therein lies the problem. To unambiguously define a variable it must be measured in isolation, i.e., in a context in which the variable is uncoupled from the remainder of the universe. This situation can sometimes be achieved in the physical sciences (leaving quantum mechanical considerations aside), but not so in the social and life sciences. Thus, one must *assume* that the operational definition of a variable is sufficient for the purposes of using the concept in the formulation of a model. This assumption presumes that the interaction of the variable with other "operationally defined" variables constituting the system is sufficiently weak that for some specified conditions the interactions may be neglected. In the physical sciences one has come to call such effects "weak interactions" and perturbation theories have been developed to describe successively stronger interactions between a variable and the physical system of interest. Not only is there no *a priori* reason why this should be true in general, but in point of fact there is a great deal of experimental evidence that it is not true.

Consider the simple problem of measuring the physical dimensions of a tube, when that tube is part of a complex physiological structure such as the lung or the cardiovascular system. Classical measuring theory tells us how we should proceed. After all, the diameter of the tube is just proportional to a standard unit of length with which the measurement is taken. Isn't it? The answer to this question may be no. The length of a cord or a tube is not necessarily given by the classical result. In a number of physical and biomedical systems there may in fact be no fundamental scale of length (be it distance or time) with which to measure the properties of the system, the length may depend on how we measure it. The experimental evidence for and implications of this remark are presented in Chapter 2 where we introduce and discuss the concept of a fractal (Mandelbrot, 1977, 1982; West and Goldberger, 1987).

In 1733 Jonathan Swift wrote:

> So, Nat'ralist observe, a Flea
> Hath smaller Fleas that on him prey,
> And these have smaller Fleas to bit 'em,
> And so proceed *ad infinitum*.

and some 129 years later de Morgan modified these verses to

> Great fleas have little fleas
> upon their backs to bite 'em
> and little fleas have lesser fleas,
> and so *ad infinitum*.

These couplets capture an essential feature of what is now one of the most exciting concepts in the physical and biological sciences. This is the notion that the dynamical activity we observe in many natural phenomena is related from one level to the next by means of a scaling relation. These poets observed a self-similarity between scales, small versions of what is observed on the largest scales repeat in an ever decreasing cascade of activity at smaller and smaller scales. Processes possessing this characteristic are known as *fractals*. There is no simple compact definitions of a fractal, but all attempts at one incorporates the idea that the whole is made up of parts similar to the whole in some way. For example, those processes described by fractal time manifest their scale invariance through their spectra in which the various frequencies contributing to the dynamics are tied together through an inverse power law of the form $1/f^{\alpha}$, where f is the frequency and α is a positive constant related to the fractal dimension, a fractal dimension in general being non-integer.

1.2 How Do Nonlinearities Change Our View?

Mathematical models of biological phenomena and those developed for biomedical applications have traditionally relied on the paradigm of classical physics. The potency of this paradigm lies in the ability of physics to relate cause and effect in physical phenomena, and thereby to make predictions. Not all natural phenomena are predictable, however. As we mentioned earlier, weather is an example of a physical phenomena which remains unpredictable. Scientists believe that they understand how to construct the basic equations of motion governing the weather, and to a greater or lesser extent they understand how to solve these equations. But even with that the weather remains an enigma; predictions can only be made in terms of probabilities (Lorenz, 1963). The vulnerability of the traditional physics paradigm is revealed in that these phenomena do not display a clear cause/effect relation. A slight perturbation in the equations of motion can generate an unpredicatably large effect. Thus we say that the underlying process is random and that the equations of motion are stochastic. A great deal of scientific effort has gone into making this view consistent with the idea that the random elements in the description would disappear if sufficient information were available about the initial state of the system, so that *in principle* the evolution of the system is predictable.

As Crutchfield, Farmer, Packard and Shaw (1987) point out, this viewpoint has been altered by the discovery that simple deterministic systems with only a few degrees of freedom can generate random behavior. They emphasize that the random aspect is fundamental to the system dynamics and gathering more information will not reduce the degree of uncertainty. Randomness generated in this way is now called *chaos*. The distinction between the ''traditional'' view and the ''modern'' view of randomness is captured in the quotations from Pierre Simon de Laplace and Henri Poincaré:

Laplace, 1776
''The present state of the system of nature is evidently a consequence of what it was in the preceding moment, and if we conceive of an intelligence which at a given instant comprehends all the relations of the entities of this universe, it could state the respective positions, motions, and general affects of all these entities at any time in the past or future.''

"Physical astronomy, the branch of knowledge which does the greatest honor to the human mind, gives us an idea, albeit imperfect, of what such an intelligence would be. The simplicity of the law by which the celestial bodies move, and the relations of their masses and distances, permit analysis to follow their motions up to a certain point; and in order to determine the state of the system of these great bodies in past or future centuries, it suffices for the mathematician that their position and their velocity be given by observation for any moment in time. Man owes that advantage to the power of the instrument he employs, and to the small number of relations that it embraces in its calculations. But ignorance of the different causes involved in the productions of events, as well as their complexity, taken together with the imperfection of analysis, prevents our reaching the same certainty about the vast majority of phenomena. Thus there are things that are uncertain for us, things more or less probable, and we seek to compensate for the impossibility of knowing them by determining their different degrees of likelihood. So it is that we owe to the weakness of the human mind one of the most delicate and ingenious of mathematical theories, the science of chance or probability."

Poincaré 1903
"A very small cause which escapes our notice determines a considerable effect that we cannot fail to see, and then we say that the effect is due to chance. If we knew exactly the laws of nature and the situation of the universe at the initial moment, we could predict exactly the situation of that same universe at a succeeding moment. But even if it were the case that the natural laws had no longer any secret for us, we could still only know the initial situation *approximately*. If that enabled us to predict the succeeding situation with *the same approximation*, that is all we require, and we should say that the phenomenon had been predicted, that it is governed by laws. But it is not always so; it may happen that small differences in the initial conditions produce very great ones in the final phenomena. A small error in the former will produce an enormous error in the latter. Prediction becomes impossible, and we have the fortuitous phenomenon."

Laplace believed in strict determinism and to his mind this implied complete predictability. Uncertainty for him is a consequence of imprecise knowledge, so that probability theory is necessitated by incomplete and imperfect observations. Poincaré on the other hand sees an intrinsic inability to make predictions due to a sensitive dependence of the evolution of the system on the initial state of the system. This sensitivity arises from an intrinsic instability of the system.

Recall the notion of a phase space and of a trajectory to describe the dynamics of a system. Each choice of an initial state produces a different trajectory. If however there is a limiting set in phase space to which all trajectories are drawn after a sufficiently long time, we say that the system dynamics are described by an attractor. The attractor is the geometric limiting set on which all the trajectories eventually find themselves, i.e. the set of points in phase space to which the trajectories are attracted. Attractors come in many shapes and sizes, but they all have the property of occupying a finite volume of phase space. Initial points off the attractor initiate trajectories that are drawn to it if they lie in the attractor's *basin of attraction*. As a system evolves it sweeps through the attractor, going through some regions rather rapidly and others quite slowly, but always staying on the attractor. Whether or not the system is chaotic is determined by how two initially adjacent trajectories cover the attractor over time. As Poincaré stated, a small change in the initial separation (error) of any two trajectories will produce an enormous change in their final separation (error). The question is how this separation is accomplished on an attractor of finite size. The answer has to do with the layered structure necessary for an attractor to be chaotic.

Rössler (1978) described chaos as resulting from the geometric operations of stretching and folding often called the Baker's transformation. The conceptual baker in this transformation takes some dough and rolls it out on a floured bread board. When thin enough he folds the dough back onto itself and rolls it out again. To transform this image into a mathematically precise statement we assume that the baker rolls out the dough until it is twice as long as it is wide (the width remains constant during this operation) and then folds the extended piece back reforming the initial square. For a cleaner image we may assume that the baker cuts the dough before neatly placing the one piece atop the other. Arnol'd gave a memorable image of this process using the image of the head of a cat (cf. Arnol'd and Avery, 1968). In Figure 1.2.1 a cross section of the square of dough is shown with the head of cat inscribed. After the first rolling operation the head is flattened and stretched, i.e., it becomes half its height and twice its length. It is then cut in the center and the segment of dough to the right is set above the one on the left to reform the initial square. The operation is repeated again and we see that at the bottom the cat's head is now embedded in four layers of dough., Even after two of these transformations the cat's head is clearly decimated. After twenty stages of transformation the head will be distributed across 10^6 layers of dough – not easy to identify. As so charmingly put by Ekeland (1988): "Arnol'd's cat has melted into the square, gradually disappearing from sight like the Cheshire cat in Wonderland."

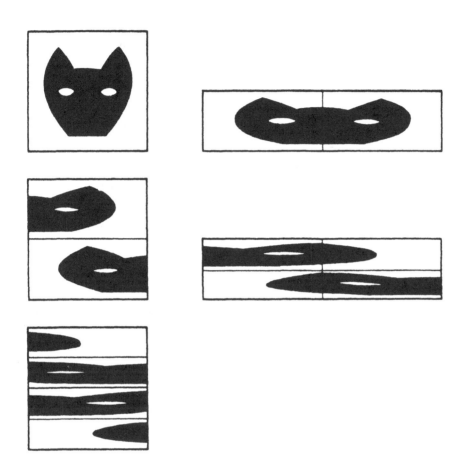

Figure 1.2.1.   Arnol'd's cat being decimated by the Baker's Transformation.

Two initially nearby orbits cannot rapidly separate forever on a finite attractor, therefore the attractor must eventually fold over onto itself. Once folded the attractor is again stretched and folded again. This process is repeated over and over yielding an attractor structure with an infinite number of layers to be traversed by the various trajectories. The infinite richness of the attractor structure affords ample opportunity for trajectories to diverge and follow increasingly different paths. The finite size of the attractor insures that these diverging trajectories will eventually pass close to one another again, albeit on different layers of the attractor. Crutchfield et al. (1987) visualize these orbits on a chaotic attractor as being shuffled by this process, much as a deck of cards is shuffled by a dealer (see also Ekeland, 1988). Thus the randomness of the chaotic orbits is a consequence of this shuffling process. We will see subsequently that this process of stretching and folding creates folds within folds ad infinitum, resulting in a fractal structure in phase space. We discuss the fractal concept in Chapter 2; the essential fractal feature of interest here is that the greater the magnification of a region of the attractor, the greater the degree of detail that is revealed.

There are a number of measures of the degree of chaos of these attractors. One is its "dimension", integer values of the dimension indicates a simple attractor, a non-integer dimension indicates a chaotic attractor in phase space. Part of our task here is to understand the various definitions of dimension and how each of them can be realized from experimental data sets. For this reason we devote a great deal of space to a discussion of dimension in Chapter 2. A large part of this discussion centers around static physiological structure such as the lung which here serves as a paradigm of physiological complexity. If we understand the general idea of the dimension of a static structure, it will make the interpretation of the non-integer dimension of a dynamic process that much easier. In particular this geometric interpretation of a fractal is important because the attractor set in phase space is just such a static structure.

A second measure of the degree of irregularity generated by a chaotic attractor is the "entropy" of the motion. The entropy is interpreted by Crutchfield et al. (1987) as the average rate of stretching and folding of the attractor, or alternatively, as the average rate at which information is generated. The application of the information concept in the dynamic systems context has been championed by Shaw (1981,1984) and Nicolis (1985,1986). One can view the preparation of the initial state of the system as initializing a certain amount of information. The more precisely the initial state can be specified, the more information one has available. This corresponds to localizing the initial state of the system in phase space, the amount of information is inversely proportional to the volume of state space localized by measurement. In a regular attractor, trajectories initiated in a given local volume stay near to one another as the system evolves, so the initial information is preserved in time and no new information is generated. Thus the initial information can be used to predict the final state of the system. In a chaotic attractor the stretching and folding operations smear out the initial volume, thereby destroying the initial information as the system evolves and the dynamics create new information. Thus the initial uncertainty in the specification of the system is eventually smeared out over the entire attractor and all predictive power is lost, i.e., *all causal connection between the present and the future is lost*. This is referred to as sensitive dependence on initial conditions.

Let us denote the region of phase space as initially occupied by V_i (initial volume) and the final region by V_f. The change in the observable information I is then (Shaw, 1981; Nicolis and Tsuda, 1985)

$$\delta I = \log_2 \frac{V_f}{V_i} \quad . \tag{1.2.1}$$

The rate of information creation or dissipation is given by

$$\frac{dI}{dt} = \frac{1}{V}\frac{dV}{dt} \quad . \tag{1.2.2}$$

In non-chaotic systems, the sensitivity of the flow in the initial conditions grows with time at most as a polynomial, e.g., let $\omega(t)$ be the number of distinguishable states so that

$$\omega(t) \sim t^n \tag{1.2.3}$$

since $V_f/V_i = \omega_f/\omega_i$ we have (Shaw 1981)

$$\frac{dI}{dt} \sim \frac{n}{t} \quad . \tag{1.2.4}$$

Thus the rate of information generation converges to zero as $t \to \infty$ and the final state is predictable from the initial information. On the other hand, in chaotic systems the sensitivity of the flow on initial conditions grow exponentially with time,

$$\omega(t) \sim e^{nt} \tag{1.2.5}$$

so that

$$\frac{dI}{dt} \sim n \quad . \tag{1.2.6}$$

This latter system is therefore a continuous source of information, the attractor itself generates the information independently of the initial conditions. This property of chaotic dynamic systems was used by Nicolis and Tsuda (1985) to model cognitive systems. The concepts from chaotic attractors are used for information processing in neurophysiology, cognitive psychology and perception (Nicolis, 1986). To pursue these latter applications in any detail would take up too far afield, but we continue to mention the existence of such applications where appropriate.

The final measure of the degree of chaos associated with an attractor with which we will be concerned is the set of Lyapunov exponents. These exponents quantify the average exponential convergence or divergence of nearby trajectories in the phase space of the dynamical systems. Wolf, Swift, Swinney and Vastano (1985) believe the spectrum of Lyapunov exponents provides the most complete qualitative and quantitative characterization of chaotic behavior. A system with one or more positive Lyapunov exponents is defined to be chaotic. The local stability properties of a system are determined by its response to perturbations; along certain directions the response can be stable whereas along others it can be unstable. If we consider a d-dimensional sphere of initial conditions and follow the evolution of this sphere in time, then in some directions the sphere will contract, whereas in others it will expand, thereby forming a d-dimensional ellipsoid. Thus, a d-dimensional system can be characterized by d exponents where the jth Lyapunov exponent quantifies the expansion or contraction of the flow along the jth ellipsoidal principal axis. The sum of the Lyapunov exponents is the average divergence, which for a dissipative system (possessing an attractor) must always be negative.

Consider a three-dimensional phase space in which the limiting set (the attractor) can be characterized by the triple of Lyapunov exponents $(\lambda_1, \lambda_2, \lambda_3)$. The qualitative behavior of the attractor can be specified by determining the signs of the Lyapunov exponents only, i.e., $(sign\,\lambda_1, sign\,\lambda_2, sign\,\lambda_3)$. As shown in Figure 1.2.2a the triple (-,-,-) corresponds to an attracting fixed point. In each of the three directions there is an exponential contraction of trajectories, so that no matter what the initial state of the system it will eventually wind up at the fixed point. This fixed point need not be the origin, as it would be for a dissipative linear system, but can be anywhere in phase space. The

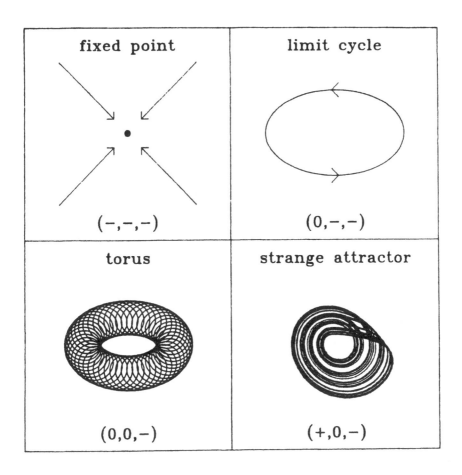

Figure 1.2.2.   Signs of Lyapunov exponents of different attractor types in a three-dimensional phase space.

arrows shown in the figure do not necessarily represent trajectories since the fixed point can be approached at any angle by the evolving nonlinear system. An attracting limit cycle is denoted by (0,-,-) in which there are two contracting directions and one that is neutrally stable. In Figure 1.2.2b we see that this attractor resembles the orbit of a van der Pol oscillator. The triple (0,0,-) has two neutral directions and one that is contracting so that the attractor is the 2-torus depicted in Figure 1.2.2c. Finally (+, 0, -) corresponds to a chaotic attractor in which the trajectories expand in one direction, are neutrally stable in another and contracting in a third. In order for the trajectories to continuously expand in one direction and yet remain on a finite attractor, the attractor must undergo stretching and folding operations in this direction. Much more will be said about this in Chapter 3.

It should be emphasized that the type of attractor describing a systems' dynamics is dependent on certain parameter values. We review the relation between parameter values and the forms of the dynamic attractor in Chapter 3. We show therein how a system can undergo transitions from simple periodic motion to apparently unorganized chaotic dynamics. It is therefore apparent that the Lyapunov exponents are dependent on these control parameters.

The notion of making a transition from periodic to chaotic dynamics lead Macky and Glass (1977) to introduce the term *dynamical disease* to denote pathological states of physiological systems over which control has been lost. Rapp, Latta, and Mees (1988) as well as Goldberger and West (1987a) make the general observation that chaotic behavior is not inevitably pathological. That is to say that, for some physiological processes, chaos may be the normal state of affairs and transitions to and from the steady state and periodic behavior may be deleterious. Experimental support for this latter point of view will be presented herein.

1.3   Summary

Nonlinear dynamical systems theory (NDST) emerged from the fusion of two classical areas of mathematics: topology and the theory of differential equations. The importance of NDST to the experimental sciences lies in its capacity to quantitatively characterize complex dynamical behavior. In this monograph we review how dynamical systems theory is applied in various biomedical contexts. One way in which it is applied is in the construction of simple dynamical models that give rise to solutions that resembles the time series data observed experimentally. Another way in which it is applied is through the development of data processing algorithms that capture the essential features of the dynamics of the system, such as its degree of irregularity and the structure of the attractor on which the system's dynamics takes place. It is obvious that the theory of differential equations is useful because it enables us to construct the dynamic equations that describe the evolution of the biomedical system of interest. Topology is of value here because it allows us to determine the unique geometrical properties of the resulting dynamic attractors. The degree of irregularity or randomness of measured time series is closely related to the geometrical structure of the underlying attractor and so we devote Chapter 2 to a new understanding of geometry.

Euclidean geometry is concerned with the understanding of straight lines and regular forms and it is assumed that the world consists of continuous smooth curves in spaces of integer dimension. When we look at billowing cumulus clouds, trees of all kinds, coral formations and coastlines we observe that the notions of classical geometry are inadequate to describe them. Detail does *not* become less and less important as regions of these various structures are magnified, but perversely more and more detail is revealed at each level of magnification. The rich texture of these structures is characteristic of fractals. In Chapter 2 we show that a fractal structure is not smooth and homogeneous, and that the smaller-scale structure is similar to the large-scale form. What makes such a structure different from what we usually experience is that there is no characteristic length scale. The more traditional concepts of scaling (Nielsen, 1984; MacDonald, 1983) are quite familiar in biology, but the application of fractal concepts are rather new. As we show, lungs, hearts and many other anatomical structures are fractal-like.

It is not only static structures that have fractal properties but dynamics processes as well. We examine how the concept of a fractal or fractional dimension can be applied to time series resulting from physiological processes. A dynamic fractal process is one that cannot be characterized by a single scale of time, analogous to a fractal structure like the lung, which is shown in Chapter 2 not to have a characteristic scale of length. Instead, fractal processes have many component frequencies, ie. they are characterized by a broad band spectrum. Fractal dynamics can be detected by analyzing the time series using spectral techniques often resulting in inverse power-law spectra. This kind of spectrum suggests that the processes that regulate different complex physiological systems over time are also governed by fractal scaling mechanisms (West and Goldberger, 1987).

The dynamics of biological systems are considered in Chapter 3. There are a large number of rather sophisticated mathematical concepts that must be developed for latter use and this is done through various worked out examples. The whole idea of modeling physiological systems by continuous differential equations is discussed in the context of bio-oscillators, which are nonlinear oscillators capable of spontaneous excitation, and strange attractors, which are sets of dissipative nonlinear equations capable of generating áperiodic time series. The distinction between limit cycle attractors and strange attractors is basic to the understanding of biomedical time series data taken up in the last chapter.

Not only continuous differential equations are of interest here, but so too are discrete equations. Discrete dynamical models appear in a natural way to describe the time evolution of biosystems in which successive time intervals are distinct, e.g. to model changes in population levels between successive generations where change occurs between generations and not within a given generation. These discrete dynamical models are referred to as *mappings* and may be used directly to model the evolution of a system or they may be used in conjunction with time series data to deduce the underlying dynamical structure of a biological process. As in the continuum case the discrete dynamic equations can have both periodic and áperiodic solutions, that is to say the *maps* also generate *chaos* in certain parameter regimes. Since such physiological processes as the interbeat interval of the mammalian heart can be characterized as a mapping, that is, one beat is mapped into the next beat by the "cardiac map," it is of interest to know how the intervals between beats are related to the map. We discuss how a map can undergo a sequence of period doubling bifurcations to make a transition from a periodic to a chaotic solution. The latter solution has been used by some to describe the normal dynamic state of the human heart.

As we mentioned earlier, one indicator of the qualitative dynamics of a system, whether it is continuous or discrete, is the Lyapunov exponent. In either case its sign determines whether nearby orbits will exponentially separate from one another in time. In Chapter 3 we present the formal rules for calculating this exponent in both simple systems and for general N-dimensional maps. Of particular concern is how one relates the Lyapunov exponents to the information generated by the dynamics. This question is particularly important in biological systems because it provides one of the measures of a strange attractor. Other measures that are discussed include the power spectrum of a time series, i.e., the Fourier transform of the two-point correlation function; the correlation dimension (a bound on the fractal dimension) obtained from the two-point correlation function on a dynamical attractor; and the phase space portrait of the attractor reconstructed from the data. These latter two measures are shown to be essential in the processing of biomedical time series and interpreting the underlying dynamics generating the observed time trace.

The method of reconstructing the phase space portrait of the dynamic system using time series data was first demonstrated by Packard, et al. (1980), and was an application of the embedding theorems of Whitney (1936) and Takens (1981). Chapter 4 is devoted to the application of this technique to a number of biomedical and chemical phenomena. It has helped us to understand the dynamics of epidemics, including how chaotic attractors can explain the observed variability in certain cases without external fluctuations driving the system. In a similar way the excitability of neurons do not require membrane noise in the traditional sense to account for their fluctuations, but rather can result from chaotic response to stimulation. The first example of the application of this technique to data was to chemical reactions, such as the Belousov-Zhabotinskii reaction (see e.g. Field, 1987) and certain enzyme reactions (Olsen and Degn, 1977). Finally we discuss how chaos arises in the heart, from the excitation of aggregates of embryonic cells of chick hearts (Glass, Guevara, Shrier and Perez, 1983) to the normal beating of the human heart (Babloyantz and Destexhe, 1988).

In Chapter 4 we also review the use of the reconstruction technique on EEG time series data to help us understand the various states of variability that are so apparent in the human brain. In addition the correlation dimension is used to determine the geometrical structure of the attractor underlying the brain wave activity. First we examine normal brain wave activity and find that one can both construct the phase space portraits of the attractors and determine the fractional dimension of the attractors. A number of difficulties associated with the data processing techniques are uncovered in these analyses and ways to improve the efficiency of these methods are proposed. One result that clearly emerges from the calculations is that the dimension of the "cognitive attractor" decreases monotonically as a subject changes from quiet, awake and eyes open to deeper stages of sleep.

On the theoretical side we discuss the model of Freeman (1987) which he developed to describe the dynamics of the olfactory system in a rat. It is found that the basal olfactory EEG signal is not sinusoidal, but is irregular and aperiodic. This intrinsic unpredictability is captured by the model in that the solutions are chaotic attractors for certain classes of parameter values. These theoretical results are quite in keeping with the experimental observations of normal EEG records.

One of the more dramatic results that has been obtained in recent years is the precipitous drop in the correlation dimension of the EEG time series when an individual undergoes an epileptic seizure. The brain's attractor seems to have a dimensionality on the order of 4 or 5 in deep sleep and to have the much lower dimensionality of approximately 2 in the epileptic state. This sudden drop in dimensionality was successfully captured in the Freeman model in which he calculated the EEG time series for a rat undergoing a seizure.

We show studies that demonstrate there to be a clear progression of the dimension magnitude from quiet, awake, eyes closed (approximately 5) to quiet, awake, eyes closed using verbal memory (approximately 6.3). In addition to this distinct ordering of the mental task performed and the magnitude of the dimension, there is a decrease in the variance of the dimension as the state of the brain changes from no task to one involving cognitive activity. The trend in these data supports the hypothesis that the dimension of the EEG time series is closely tied to the cognitive activity of the brain.

2. PHYSIOLOGY IN FRACTAL DIMENSIONS

Although it is our intent to understand certain of the dynamics features contained in biomedical time series data using the methods of nonlinear data analysis, we find it useful to introduce a number of the fundamental concepts through an investigation of more familiar static physiological structures. This approach highlights the new insights that can be gained by the application of such concepts as self-similarity, fractals, renormalization group relations and power-law distributions to physiology.

The complex interrelationship between biological development, form and function are evident in many physiological structures including the finely branched bronchial tree and the ramified His-Purkinje conduction network of the heart. In the early part of this century such relations were explored in exquisite detail in the seminal work of D'Arcy Thompson (1917). It was his conviction that although biological systems evolve by rules that may be distinct from those which govern the development of physical systems, they cannot violate basic physical laws. This ideal of underlying physical constraints led to the formulation of several important scaling relations in biology-describing, for example, how proportions tend to vary as an animal grows.

Relationships that depend on scale can have profound implications for physiology. A simple example of Thompson's approach is provided by the application of engineering considerations to the determination of the maximum size of terrestrial bodies (vertebrates). The strength of a bone increases in direct proportion to its cross-sectional area (the square of its linear dimension) whereas its weight increases in proportion to its volume (the cube of its linear dimension). Thus there comes a point where a bone does not have sufficient strength to support its own weight, as first observed by Galileo Galilei in 1638. The point of collapse is given by the intersection of a quadratic and a cubic curve denoting, respectively, the strength and weight of a bone (cf. Figure 2.0.1). A second example, which is actually a variant of the first, recognizes that mass increases as the cube of its linear dimension, but the surface area increases only as the square. According to this principle, if one species is twice as tall as another, it is likely to be eight times heavier but to have only four times as much surface area. This tells us immediately that the larger plants and animals must compensate for their bulk; respiration depends on surface area for the exchange of gases as does cooling by evaporation from the skin and nutrition by absorption through membranes. One way to add surface to

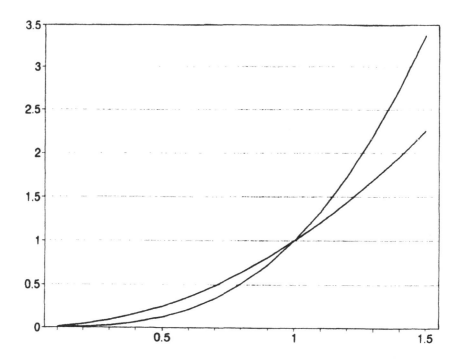

Figure 2.0.1. The strength of a bone increases as $S \sim l^2$ whereas its weight increases as $W \sim l^3$, the intersection of the two curves yields $S = W$. Beyond this point the structure becomes unstable.

a given volume is to make the exterior more irregular, as with branches and leaves on trees; another is to hollow out the interior as with some cheeses. The human lung, with 300 million air sacs, approaches the more favorable ratio of surface to volume enjoyed by our evolutionary ancestors, the single-celled microbes.

It is at this last point that the classical concepts of scaling developed by Thompson and others fails. They are not capable of accounting for the irregular surfaces and structures seen in the heart, lung, intestine, and brain. The classical approach relied on the assumption that biological processes like their physical counterparts, are continuous, homogeneous, and regular. Observations and experiment however, suggest the opposite. Most biological systems, and many physical ones, are discontinuous, inhomogeneous, and irregular and are necessarily this way in order to perform a particular function. It has long been recognized that the characterization of these kinds of systems requires new models. In this chapter we discuss how the related concepts of *fractals*, nonanalytic mathematical functions, and renormalization group transformations provide novel approaches to the study of physiological form and function.

Perhaps the most compelling feature of all physiological systems is their complexity. Capturing the richness of physiological structure and function in a single model presents one of the major challenges of modern biology. On a static (structural) level, the bronchial system of the lung serves as a useful paradigm for such anatomic complexity. One sees in this tree-like network a complicated hierarchy of airways, beginning with the trachea and branching down on an increasingly smaller scale to the level of tiny tubes called bronchioles (see Figure 2.0.2). We return to the pulmonary tree in considerable detail subsequently, but an essential prelude to a *quantitative* analysis of this kind of complex structure is an appreciation for its *qualitative* features.

Any successful model of pulmonary structure must account not only for the details of *microscopic* (small scale) measurements, but also for the global organization of these smaller units. It is the *macroscopic* (large scale) structure we observe with the unaided eye, and initially one is struck with at least two features of bronchial architecture. The

24

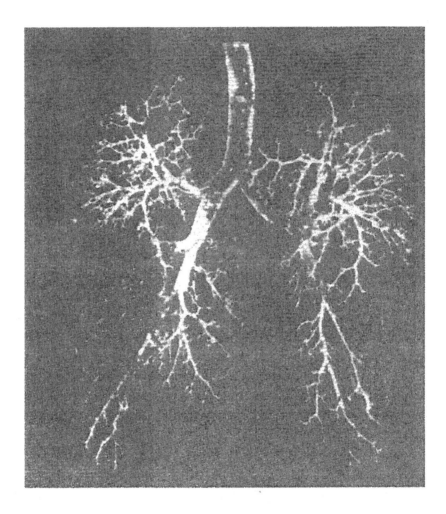

Figure 2.0.2. The photograph shows a plastic cast of the human bronchial tree, from the
trachea to the terminal bronchioles. The mammalian lung, has long been a
paradigm of natural complexity, challenging scientists to reduce its structure and growth to simple rules. (From West and Goldberger, 1987.)

first is the extreme variability of tube lengths and diameters and the second is the high level of organization. The first of these paradoxical observations results from the fact that the branching of a given airway is not uniform: the two tubes emerging from a given branching vertex are not of equal length. One numbering convention is to label successive bifurcations of the bronchial tree by generation number. The first generation of tubes is comprised of just two members, the left and right mainstem bronchi. The second generation consists of four tubes, and so forth (cf. Figure 2.0.3). Clearly from one generation to the next the tubes vary, tending to get smaller and smaller in both length and diameter. But the variability of the lung is not restricted to comparisons *between* generations. As one can see, the tubes also vary markedly in size within any given generation.

The second predominant impression of the lung which seems to contradict this initial sense of variability, is that of *organization*. The bronchial tree, for all its asymmetries, is clearly constructed along some ordering principle(s). There appear to be some pattern or patterns underlying the irregularity of the multiple tube sizes. It is this paradoxical combination of variability and order which must emerge from any successful model of bronchial architecture. Indeed, we will be forced to reject as "unphysiologic" any model which fails to encompass these two features. Further, we find that the fractal concept is quite useful in modeling the observed variability of the lung (West, Bhargava and Goldberger, 1986).

The question of anatomic regularity and variability is only one aspect of the general problem of physiologic complexity. We also seek to understand certain features of *dynamical* complexity, so that in addition to their static structure, the real time functioning of physiological systems can be explained. We postpone this aspect of our discussion to the next section where we consider dynamic processes in general. Measurement of physiological systems under "free-running" circumstances gives rise to data sets that are notable for their erratic variations. The statistical techniques required for the analysis of such data sets are formidable. In dealing with healthy physiological systems, therefore, the tradition is to restrict the experiment sufficiently so that this "noise" is filtered from the data. Such carefully controlled observations, while useful in dissecting selected aspects of physiological behavior, do have a major shortcoming: they do not allow a general, quantitative description of healthy function with its potentially unbounded number of degrees of freedom.

26

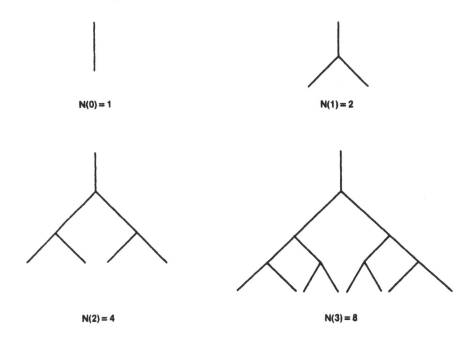

Figure 2.0.3. Here we depict a simple dichotomous network where z denotes the generation number and $N(z)$ is the number of branches in the zth generation.

If, for example, you feel your pulse while resting, your heart rate appears relatively regular. However, if you were to record the activity of your heart during a vigorous day's activity, a far different impression of the normal heartbeat would be obtained. Instead of exclusively observing some apparently calm steady state, you would record periods of sharp fluctuations interspersed between these apparently regular intervals (see Figure 2.0.4).

Just as we suggested that any useful model of lung anatomy would have to explain both its variability and order, we can now insist on the same criteria for judging the success of any model of cardiovascular dynamics. Our understanding of heart rate variability must account for the fluctuations seen in the free-running, "non-equilibrium," *healthy* state of the heart.

Over the past several years, in collaboration with our colleagues Drs. Ary Goldberger, Valmik Bhargava and Arnold Mandell of the University of California, San Diego, we have developed quantitative models which we hope will suggest a mechanism for the "organized variability" inherent in physiological structure and function. The essential concept underlying this kind of constrained randomness is that of *scaling* (Mandell, Russo and Knapp, 1982; West, 1985). The general notion of scaling, as we have already mentioned, is well established in biology via the work of D'Arcy Thompson and others (MacDonald, 1983; Schmidt-Nielsen, 1984; Goldberger, Bhargava, West and Mandell, 1985; West, 1988). However, the scaling mechanism we will subsequently discuss adds to these traditional theories a few wrinkles which are as yet unfamiliar to most physiologists. At the same time, in the non-biological sciences, these new models of scaling have already emerged as an important strategy in understanding a variety of complex systems. The "new scaling," for example, appears in related guise in the description of a ubiquitous class of irregular structures called *fractals*, in the theory of critical phenomena (renormalization group theory), and in the "chaotic" dynamics of nonlinear systems.

The fractal concept developed in recent years by Mandelbrot (1977, 1982) arises in three distinct, but related guises. (From his definition of the term in 1977 there has grown an industry of publication on fractals, probably exceeding a thousand journal articles per year.) The first context in which we find fractals deals with complex

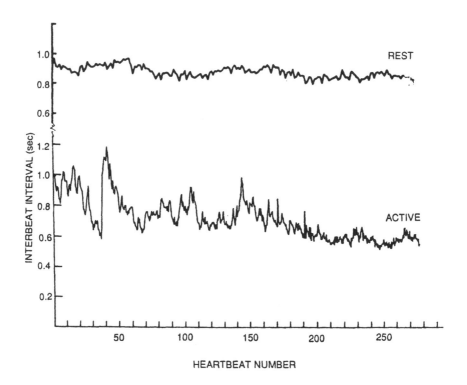

Figure 2.0.4. The contrast in the heart rate variability for a healthy individual between the resting state and that of normal activity is quite dramatic. Any model that is to successfully describe cardiovascular dynamics must be able to explain both the order of the resting state and the variability of the active state.

geometric forms. A fractal structure is not smooth and homogeneous but rather when examined with stronger and stronger magnifying lenses, reveals greater and greater levels of detail. Many objects in nature, including trees, coral formations, cumulus clouds and coastlines are fractal. As we have mentioned and will later show, lungs, hearts, and many other anatomic structures also possess fractal properties (West et al., 1986; Goldberger et al., 1985). A second guise in which one finds fractals has to do with the statistical properties of a process. Here it is the statistics that are inhomogeneous and irregular rather than smooth. A fractal statistical process is one in which there is a statistical rather a geometrical sameness to the process at all levels of magnification. Thus just as the geometrical structure satisfies a scaling relation so too does the stochastic process. The extreme variability in the sizes of airways "within" a given generation of the lung is an example of such statistics (West, 1987, 1988). The final context in which fractals are observed involves time and is related to dynamical processes. An example is the voltage measured at the myocardium arising from the cardiac pulses emerging from the His-Purkinje condition system of the heart (Goldberger et al., 1985). Again, more and more structure is revealed in the voltage time series as the scale of observation is reduced. Furthermore, the smaller-scale structure is similar to the larger scale form. In this latter situation there is no characteristic time scale in the time series because the structure of the conduction system is a fractal tree. Here we see one of the connections between geometric structure and dynamics.

In applying the new scaling ideas to physiology we have seen that irregularity, when admitted as fundamental rather than treated as a pathological deviation from some classical ideal, can paradoxically suggest a more powerful unifying theory. To describe the advantage of the new concepts we must first review some classical theories of scaling.

2.1 The Principle of Similitude

The concept of *similitude* or sameness emerges in a general way as the central theme in D'Arcy Thompson's studies of biological structure and function. A compelling illustration of this principle is provided by the geometry of spiral sea shells, such as the nautilus shown in Figure 2.1.1. Based on carefully compiled measurements, Thompson described that the nautilus followed a pattern originally described by René Descartes in 1683 as the *equiangular spiral* and subsequently by Jakob Bernoulli as the *logarithmic spiral*. Bernoulli, in fact, was so taken with this figure that he called it *spira mirabilis*

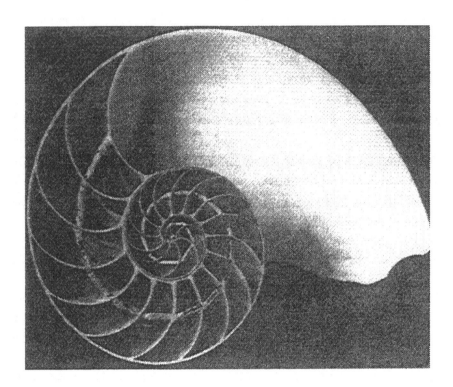

Figure 2.1.1.   The principle of similitude is exemplified in the logarithmic, or equiangular, spiral (in polar coordinates, $\log r = k\theta$). An organism growing in
such a spiral retains its original proportions while its size increases, as can
be seen in the shell of the pearly nautilus (*Nautilus Pompilius*, cross section). (From West and Goldberger, 1987.)

and requested that it be inscribed on his tombstone. The special feature of this type of spiral which has intrigued mathematicians and which became the central theme of Thompson's biological modeling is the similitude principle. As D'Arcy Thompson (1917) wrote:

"In the growth of a shell, we can conceive no simpler law than this, namely that it shall widen and lengthen in the same unvarying proportions: and this simplest of laws is that which nature tends to follow. The shell, like the creature within it, grows in size *but does not change its shape* and the existence of this constant relativity of growth, or constant similarity of form, is of the essence, and may be made the basis of a definition, of the equiangular spiral."

This spiral-shape is not restricted to the nautilus but was described by Thompson in many other shells. However it seems likely that the shell-like structure in the inner ear, the cochlea (from the greek word for "snail"), also follows the design of the logarithmic spiral. Its relevance to physiology has never been pursued to any great extent. The ability to preserve basic proportions is remarkable; the lung, by contrast, seems riddled with structural variations.

In 1915, two years prior to D'Arcy Thompson's work *On Growth and Form* a German physiologist, Fritz Rohrer, reported his investigations on scaling in the bronchial tree. Rohrer reviewed the properties of the flow of a Newtonian fluid in systems of pipes of varying lengths and cross-sectional areas arranged in cascades of different kinds. His purpose was to determine the properties of the flow in branched systems and from this theoretical reasoning to derive formulae for the average length and diameter of a conduit as a function of the stage (generation z) of a sequence of branches. He explored a number of assumptions regarding the scaling properties of one branch to the next in a sequence; for example, if there is a scaling only in length but not diameter, or if there is equal scaling in length and diameter, and so on. Each of his assumed properties led to different scaling relations between the flow at successive generations of the branching system of pipes. Although much of the data could be connected with different assumptions, no single set of assumed properties was recognized at that time as being clearly superior to the others. (In Figure 2.1.2 is depicted an idealized version of Rohrer's model of the lung.)

32

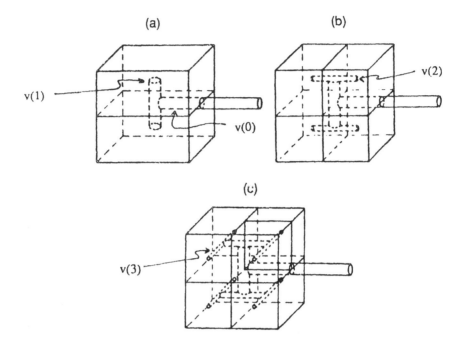

Figure 2.1.2. In this idealized sketch the total volume of the lung is viewed as a cube.
The intent is to subdivide the cube into smaller cubes in such a way that
each subcube is supplied by an airway. In (a) the initial volume of the airway bifurcates and supplies each side of the split cube with a new airway
of volume $v(1)$. Each of these new airways bifurcates to supply the air into
new additional cubes shown in (b) with new conduits of volume $v(2)$,
which in turn bifurcate into airways of volume $v(3)$ as shown in (c). This
bifurcation process is repeated until each small cube is penetrated by the
terminus of an airway.

Following Rohrer, if we denote the generation index by z, let us assume that the average length $l(z)$ of a conduit is proportional to its average diameter $d(z)$ so that the volume of an airway is $v(z) = \pi l(z) d^2(z)/4 \propto d^3(z)$. Further, if the diameter scales as $d(z) = q\, d(z-1)$ between successive generations, then the volume scales as $v(z) \propto q^3 d^3(z) = \cdots = q^{3z} v(0)$ where $v(0)$ is the volume of the airway at the $z = 0$ generation and q is a constant. For a homogeneous dichotomous branching process the volume in one generation is divided equally between the two branches $n(z)$ in the next generation. Thus, $v(z) = v(z-1)/2$ and since in this model the total volume is assumed to be constant, the number of branches must double between generations, $n(z) = 2n(z-1)$ so that the total volume $n(z)v(z) = n(z-1)v(z-1)$ remains constant on the average. Therefore the constant q is given by $1/2^{1/3}$ and the average diameter decreases exponentially with generation number, $d(z) = d(0) \exp[-z \ln(2)/3]$ where $d(0)$ is the diameter of the trachea.

The next major attempt to apply scaling concepts to the understanding of the respiratory system was made in the early sixties by Ewald Weibel and Domingo Gomez (1962). The intent of their investigation was to demonstrate the existence of fundamental relations between the size and number of lung structures. They considered the conductive airways as a dichotomous branching process, so if again z denotes the generation index and $n(z)$ denotes the number of branches in the zth generation, then $n(z) = qn(z-1)$, where q is a scaling parameter. This functional equation relating the number of branches at successive generations has the solution $n(z) = q^z$, which since $q^z = \exp(z \ln q)$ indicates that the number of airways increases exponentially with generation number at a rate given by $\ln(q)$. This solution corresponds to having only a single conduit at the $z = 0$ generation with all conduits in each stage being of equal length. The average volume of the total airway is the same between successive generations on the average, but with significant variability due to the irregular pattern of dichotomous branching in the real lung. Weibel and Gomez comment that the linear dimension of the tubes in each generation do not have a fixed value, but rather, show a distribution about some average. This variability was neglected in their theoretical analysis since it was the first attempt to capture the systematic variation in the linear dimension of the airways from generation to generation, although it was accounted for in their data analysis. Their formal results are contained in the earlier work of Rohrer if one interprets the fixed values of lengths and diameters at each generation used by him as the average values used by Weibel and Gomez.

34

Thus the human lung has two dominant features, irregularity and richness of structure along with organization. Both these characteristics are required to perform the gas exchange function for which the lung is designed. As the bronchial tree branches out, its tubes decrease in size. The *classical theory* of scaling predicts that their diameters should decrease by about the same ratio from one generation to the next. If the ratio were 1/2, for example, the relative diameters of the tubes would be 1/2, 1/4, 1/8 and so on – an exponential decline. Weibel and Gomez measured the tube diameters for 22 branchings of the bronchial tree. On semi-log graph paper the scaling prediction is that the data should lie along a straight line (cf. Figure 2.1.3).

Theodore Wilson (1965) subsequently offered an explanation for the proposed exponential decrease in the average diameter of a bronchial tube with generation number by demonstrating that this is the functional form for which a gas of a given composition can be provided to the alveoli with minimum metabolism or entropy production in the respiratory musculature. His hypothesis was that the characteristics of the design of biological systems take values for which a given function can be accomplished with minimum total entrophy production. This principle was articulated in great detail somewhat later by Glansdorf and Prigogine (1971) in a much broader physical context that includes biological systems as a special application. It is also significant that the same scaling result obtained for the diameter of the bronchial airways was also obtained by Rashevsky (1960) in his study of the arterial system in which he applied a somewhat related general principle. Rather than minimum entropy production Rashevsky believed that the optimal design to accomplish a set of prescribed functions for an organism is attained with a minimum of material used and energy expended. Each of these principles takes the form of minimizing the variation of the appropriate quantity between successive generations. The relative merits of which quantity is to be minimized and why this is a reasonable modeling strategy will not be taken up here, but rather we stress that the anatomic data apparently suggest an underlying principle that guides the morphogenesis of the bronchial tree. We return to the question of the possible relation between scaling and morphogenesis in due course.

Note that the analyses up to this point are consistent with the data for ten generations of the bronchial tree. However, when we examine Weibel and Gomez's data for the entire span of the bronchial tree data (more than twenty generations) a remarkable systematic deviation from the exponential behavior found above appears

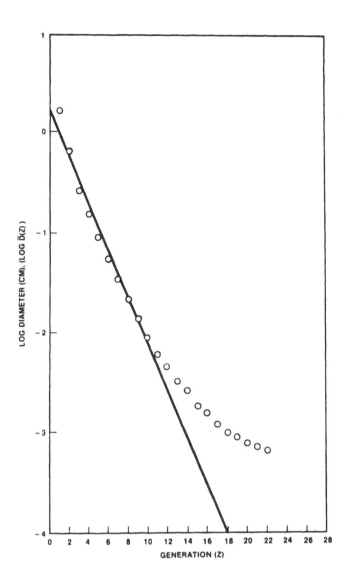

Figure 2.1.3. The human lung cast data of Weibel and Gomez for 23 generations are indicated by the circles and the prediction using the exponential form for the average diameter is given by the straight line. The fit is quite good until $z = 10$, after which there is a systematic deviation of the anatomic data from the theoretical curve. (From West et al., 1985.)

(see Figure 2.1.3). Weibel and Gomez attributed this deviation to a change in the flow mechanism in the bronchial tree from that of minimum resistance to that of molecular diffusion. We contend that the observed change in the average diameter can equally well be explained without recourse to such a change in flow properties. Recall that the arguments we have reviewed neglects the variability in the linear scales at each generation and uses only average values for the lengths and diameters. The distribution of linear scales at each generation accounts for the deviation in the average diameter from a simple exponential form. The problem is that the seemingly obvious classified scaling sets a characteristic scale size. This will clearly fail for complex systems where no characteristic scale exists. We find that the fluctuations in the linear sizes are inconsistent with simple scaling but are compatible with a more general scaling theory that satisfies a *renormalization group* property (West and Goldberger, 1987). Up to now renormalization group theory has been applied almost exclusively to the understanding of complex physical processes that are dependent on many scales (Wilson, 1979). We have introduced the relevance of this new scaling theory to physiologic variability.

The bridge between the classical scaling principles just outlined and the novel renormalization theory of scaling is the theme of *similitude*, a notion previously encountered in the discussion of the logarithmic spiral. Intuition suggests that the type of *simple* scaling function implicit in the classical notion of similitude is not adequate to describe the full range of structural variability apparent in the lung and elsewhere in physiology. Classical scaling principles, as noted before, are based on the notion that the underlying process is uniform, filling an interval in a smooth continuous fashion. In the example of the bone given by Galileo the "strength" was assumed to be uniformly distributed over the cross-sectional area with its weight having a similar uniformity. Such assumptions are not necessarily accurate. We know for example that the marrow of the bone is more porous than the periphery, so that neither the distribution of strength nor weight in a bone is uniform. We anticipate that this nonuniformity will manifest itself through a new scaling principle. The deviation of bronchial diameter measurements from the simple exponential derived by Rohrer (1915) and later by Weibel and Gomez (1962), confirm this suspicion.

The two major limitations of this classical similitude principle are: (1) it neglects the variability in linear scales at each generation and (2) it assumes the system to be *homogeneous* on scales smaller than some characteristic size. One sees however that the bronchial tube dimensions clearly show prominent fluctuations around their mean values and as you inspect the bronchial tree with greater and greater resolution, you see finer and finer details of structure. Thus, the small scale architecture of the lung, far from being homogeneous, is richly and somewhat asymmetrically structured. At the same time, there is clearly a similarity between the bronchial branchings on these smaller levels and the overall tree-like appearance.

We need to make a transition, therefore, from the notion of similitude with its implicit idea of homogeneity, to a more general concept which has come to be referred to as *self-similarity*. Is there any known scaling mechanism which will yield self-similar behavior but which is not dependent on a single scale factor? Clearly any theory of self-similar scaling which is based on a multiplicity of scales would be an attractive candidate to test physiological structures and processes which are characterized by variability and order.

2.2 Beyond Similitude; Self-Similarity, Fractals and Renormalization

In the late 19th century mathematicians addressed the problem of characterizing structures that have features of self-similarity and lack a characteristic smallest scale. Although they were not motivated by physiological concerns their work has relevance to complex physiological structures such as the lung in that as one proceeds from the trachea to the alveoli there is an average decrease in the cross-sectional area of the airway of the self-similar branches. Thus as one traverses the bronchial tree more and more tubes of smaller and smaller size appear. (Although there is a smallest size to the bronchial tubes this can be disregarded for most of the mathematical arguments to follow since it will not strongly influence the conclusions.) At any generation we can consider the distribution in tube sizes as constituting a mathematical set. To understand the bronchial tree, therefore, it is apparent that we need to have a model of a set that can be progressively "thinned out." The study of such self-similar sets was initiated in the previous century by the mathematician Georg Cantor and they now bear his name (see eg. Jourdain, 1955). Some of his ideas are surprisingly relevant to biology.

A simple example of what has come to be called a "Cantor Set" can be constructed starting from a line of unit length by systematically removing segments from specified regions of the line (see Figure 2.2.1). We indicate the set in stages, generated by removing the middle third of each line segment at the zth generation to generate the more

38

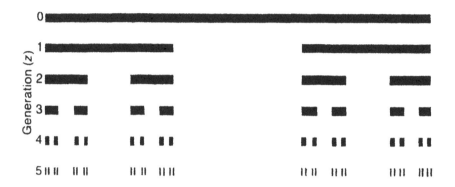

Figure 2.2.1. A Cantor set can be generated by "cutting-out" the middle third of a line segment at each generation z. The set of points remaining in the limit $z \to \infty$ is called a Cantor set. The line segments are distributed more and more sparsely with each iteration, and the resulting set of points is both discontinuous and inhomogeneous.

depleted structure at the $(z+1)st$ generation. When this procedure is taken to the limit of infinitely large z the resulting set of points is referred to as a Cantor set. It is apparent that the set of line segments becomes thinner and thinner as z is increased. It is important to visualize how the remaining line segments fill the one-dimensional line more and more sparsely with each iteration, since it is the limit distribution of points that we wish to relate to certain features of physiological structure. The line segments, like the bronchial tube sizes, become smaller and smaller, and the set of points at the limit of this trisecting operation is not continuous. How then can one characterize it?

Compared with a smooth, classical geometrical form, a fractal curve (surface) appears wrinkled. Furthermore, if the wrinkles of a fractal are examined through a microscope more wrinkles become apparent. If these wrinkles are now examined at higher magnification, still smaller wrinkles (wrinkles on wrinkles on wrinkles) appear, with seemingly endless levels of irregular structure emerging. The fractal dimension provides a measure of the degree of irregularity. A fractal as a mathematical entity has no characteristic scale size and so the emergence of irregularity proceeds to ever smaller scales. A physical fractal, on the other hand, always ends at some smallest scale as well as some largest scale and whether or not this is a useful concept depends on the size of the interval over which the process appears to be scale-free.

What then is the length of a fractal line? Clearly, there can be no simply defined length for such an irregular curve independent of the measurement scale, since the smaller the ruler used to measure it, the longer the line appears to be. For example Richardson (1960) noted that the estimated length of an irregular coastline or boundary $L(\eta)$, where η is the measuring unit, is given by

$$L(\eta) = L_0 \, \eta^{1-d} \quad . \tag{2.2.1}$$

Here L_0 is a constant with dimensions of length and d is a constant given by the slope of the linear log-log line

$$\ln L(\eta) = \ln L_0 + (1-d) \ln \eta \quad . \tag{2.2.2}$$

For a classical smooth line $d = D_T = 1$ and $L(\eta) = $ constant, independent of η where D_T is the topological dimension. For a fractal curve, such as an irregular coastline, d is the fractal dimension $d = D > D_T = 1$. In Figure 2.2.2 we see that the data for the apparent length of coastlines and boundaries fall on straight lines with slopes given by $(d-1)$.

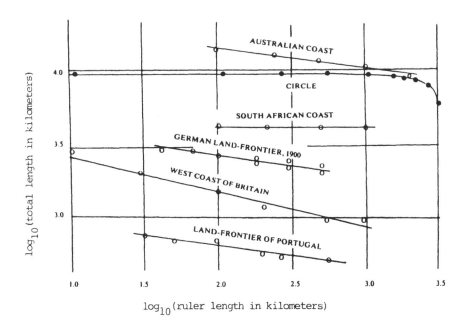

Figure 2.2.2. Fractal plots of various coastlines in which the apparent length $L(\eta)$ is graphed versus the measuring unit η: plotted as $\log_{10}$ [total length (km)] versus $\log_{10}$ [length of scales (km)]. [From Richardson (1960).]

From these data we find that $d \approx 1.3$ for the coast of Britain and $d=1$ for a circle, as expected. Thus we see that $L(\eta) \approx \eta^{-0.3} \to \infty$ as $\eta \to 0$ for a fractal curve since $(1-d) < 0$. The self-similitude of the irregular curve results in the measured length increasing without limit as the ruler size diminishes.

Mandelbrot (1982) investigated a number of curves having the above property, i.e., curves whose length depend on the ruler size. One example is the triadic Koch curve depicted in Figure 2.2.3. The construction of this curve is initiated with a line segment of unit length, $L(1) = 1$. A triangular kink is then introduced into the line resulting in four segments each of length one-third so that the total length of the *prefractal*, a term coined by Feder (1988), is $(4/3)^1$. If this process is repeated on each of the four line segments the total length of the resulting curve is $(4/3)^2$. Thus after n applications of this operation we have

$$L(\eta) = (4/3)^n \qquad (2.2.3)$$

where the length of each line segment is

$$\eta = 1/3^n \quad . \qquad (2.2.4)$$

Now the generation number n may be expressed in terms of the scale η as

$$n = -\ln \eta / \ln 3 \qquad (2.2.5)$$

so that the length of the prefractal is

$$L(\eta) = (4/3)^{-\frac{\ln \eta}{\ln 3}} = e^{-\frac{\ln \eta}{\ln 3}(\ln 4 - \ln 3)}$$

$$= \eta^{1-d} \quad . \qquad (2.2.6)$$

Comparing (2.2.6) with Richardson's equation (2.2.1) we obtain

$$d = \ln 4 / \ln 3 \approx 1.2628 \qquad (2.2.7)$$

as the fractal (Hausdorff-Besicovitch) dimension of the triadic Koch curve. Furthermore, we note that the number of line segments at the nth generation is given by $N(\eta) = 4^n = 4^{-\ln \eta / \ln 3}$ yielding

$$N(\eta) = 1/\eta^d \qquad (2.2.8)$$

as the number of line segments necessary to cover an irregular curve of fractal dimension d. [See Feder (1988) for a more complete discussion.]

42

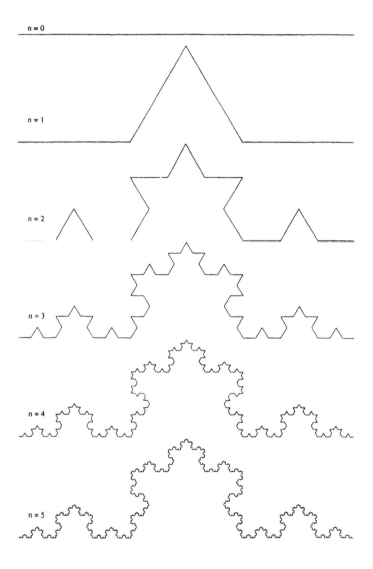

Figure 2.2.3. On a line segment of unit length a kink is formed, giving rise to four line segments, each of length 1/3. The total length of this line is 4/3. On each of these line segments a kink is formed, giving rise to 16 line segments each of length 1/9. The total length of this curve is $(4/3)^2$. This process is continued through $n = 5$ for the triadic Koch curve.

In the second decade of this century Felix Hausdorff determined that one could generally classify such a set as the one described above by means of a *fractional dimensionality* (Mandelbrot, 1977, 1982). An application of Hausdorff's reasoning can be made to the distribution of mass points in a volume of space of "radius" R, where a mass point is a convenient fiction used to denote an indivisible unit of physical mass (or probability mass) at a mathematical point in space. Any observable quantity is then built up out of large numbers of these idealized mass points. One way of picturing a distribution having a fractional dimensionality is to imagine approaching a mass distribution from a great distance. At first, the mass will seem to be in a single cluster. As one gets closer, it will be observed that the cluster is really composed of smaller clusters such that upon approaching each smaller cluster, it will seem to be composed of a set of still smaller clusters, etc. It turns out that this apparently contrived example in fact describes the distribution of stars in the heavens, and the Hausdorff dimension has been determined by astronomical observations to be approximately 1.23 (Peebles, 1980). In Figure 2.2.4 we depict how the total mass of such a cluster is related to its Hausdorff dimension.

The total mass $M(R)$ of a distribution of mass points in Figure 2.2.4a is proportional to R^d, where d is the dimension of space occupied by the masses. In the absence of other knowledge it is assumed that the point masses are uniformly distributed throughout the volume and that d is equal to the Euclidean dimension E of the space, for example in three spatial dimensions $d=E=3$. Let us suppose, however, that on closer inspection we observe that the mass points are not uniformly distributed, but instead are clumped in distinct spheres of size R/b each having a mass that is $1/a$ smaller than the total mass (cf. Figure 2.2.4b). Thus, what we had initially visualized as a beach ball filled uniformly with sand turns out to resemble one filled with basketballs, each of the basketballs being filled uniformly with sand. We now examine one of these smaller spheres (basketballs) and find that instead of the mass points being uniformly distributed in this reduced region it consists of still smaller spheres, each of radius R/b^2 and each having a mass $1/a^2$ smaller than the total mass (cf. Figure 2.2.4c). Now again the image changes so that the basketballs appear to be filled with baseballs, and each baseball is uniformly filled with sand. If we assume that this procedure of constructing spheres within spheres can be telescoped indefinitely we obtain $M(R) = \lim_{N \to \infty} [M(R/b^N) a^N]$. This relation yields a finite value for the total mass in the limit of N becoming

44

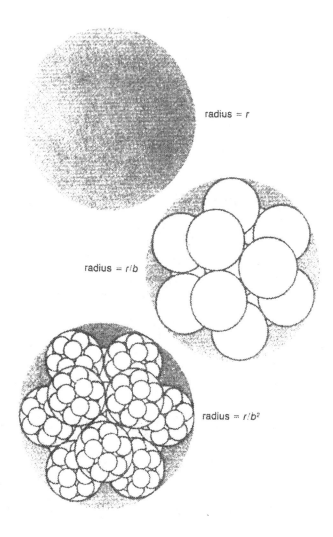

radius = r

radius = r/b

radius = r/b^2

Figure 2.2.4.   Here we schematically represent how a given mass can be nonuniformly distributed in a given volume in such a way that the volume occupied by the mass has a Hausdorff dimension $d = ln \ a / ln \ b$. The parameter b gives the scaling from the original sphere of radius r and the parameter a gives the scaling from the original total mass M assumed to be uniformly distributed in the volume r^3 to that nonuniformly distributed in the volume r^d.

infinitely large only if $d = ln\ a/ln\ b$, where d is the Hausdorff (fractional) dimension of the distribution of mass points dispersed throughout the topological volume of radius R. The index of the power-law distribution of mass points can therefore be distinct from the topological dimension of the space in which the mass is embedded, i.e., $d < E = 3$.

In a similar way the Cantor set previously discussed can be characterized by a fractional dimension d which is less than the topological dimension of the line, i.e., $d < 1$. The Hausdorff dimension, or using the term introduced into the scientist's lexicon in recent years by Benoit Mandelbrot, the *fractal dimension*, can again be specified by invoking the fiction of mass points. Imagine that the mass points are initially distributed along a line of length r. In cutting out the middle third of the line, we redistribute the mass along the remaining two segments so that the total mass of the set remains constant. At the next stage, where the middle third is cut out of each of the two line segments, we again redistribute the mass so that none is lost. We now define the parameter a as the ratio of the total mass to the mass of each segment after one trisecting operation. In this example, since each segment receives half the mass of its parent, $a = 2$. We also define a second parameter, b, as the ratio of the length of the original line to the length of each remaining segment. Since we are cutting out the middle third $b = 3$. The parameter a determines how quickly the mass is being redistributed while the parameter b gives us a comparable idea of how quickly the available space is being thinned out. The fractal dimension d of the resulting Cantor set is the ratio of logarithms $ln\ a\ /\ ln\ b$ which in our example is $ln\ 2\ /\ ln\ 3 = 0.6309$. Thus we see that the thinness of the distribution of the elements of the set is dependent on three factors. First is the dimension E of the Euclidean space in which the set is embedded. Second is the dimension d of the set itself. Third is the intuitive notion of a topological dimension. For example, a string has a topological dimension of unity because it is essentially a line regardless of how one distorts its shape and it is embedded in a Euclidean space of one higher dimension. If $d < E$, but d is greater than the topological dimension, then the set is said to be fractal and the smaller the fractal dimension the more tenuous is the set of points.

There are several ways in which one can intuitively make sense of such a fractional dimension. Note first that in this example that $1 > d > 0$ and here $E = 1$. This makes sense when one thinks of the Cantor set as a physical structure with mass: it is something less than a continuous line, yet more than a vanishing set of points. Just how much less and more is given by the ratio $ln\ a\ /\ ln\ b$. If a were equal to b, the structure would not seem to change no matter how much we magnify our original line; the mass would lump together as quickly as the length scaled down, and we would see a one-dimensional Euclidean line on every scale. If a were greater than b, however, we might see a branching or a flowering object, one that seemed to develop finer and finer structure under magnification, we might see something like the fractal trees of Figure 2.2.5, which burst out of a one-dimensional space but do not fill a two-dimensional Euclidean plane. Again, the precise character depends on the value of d: the tree at the left has a fractal dimension barely above one, and thus it is wispy and broomlike; as the dimension increases from one into two, the canopy of branches becomes more and more lush.

To explore the physiological implications of these concepts, we need to find out how such a set of points can be generated, or in the more general case how a curve with a fractal dimension can be constructed. Cantor's original interest was in the representation of functions by means of trigonometric series when the function is discontinuous or divergent at a set of points. Although he became more interested in how to choose such a set of points than in their series representation, another German mathematician, Karl Weierstrass, who was a teacher and later a colleague of Cantor, was keenly interested in the theory of functions and suggested to him a particular series representation of a function that is continuous everywhere but is differentiable nowhere.

For a function to be differentiable, one must be able to draw a well-defined, straight-line tangent to every point on the curve defined by the function. Functions describing curves for which this tangent does not exist are called nonanalytic or singular and lack certain of the properties we have come to expect from mathematical representations of physical and biological processes. For example in the empirical science of thermodynamics the derivatives of certain functions often determine the physical properties of materials such as how readily they absorb heat or how easily electricity is conducted. In some circumstances, however, the property being measured does become discontinuous as in the case of the magnetization of a piece of iron as the temperature of the sample approaches a critical value (the Curie temperature T_c). At this value of the temperature, the magnetization which was zero for $T > T_c$, jumps to a finite value and then smoothly

47

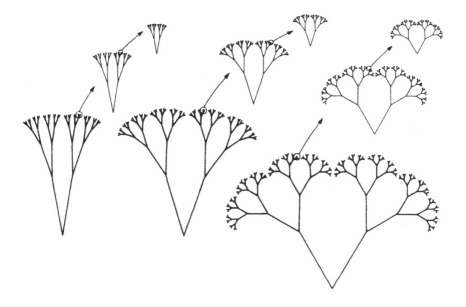

Figure 2.2.5. Fractals are a family of shapes containing infinite levels of detail, as observed in the Cantor set and in the infinitely clustering spheres. In the fractals reproduced here, the tip of each branch continues branching over many generations, on smaller and smaller scales, and each magnified, smaller-scale structure is similar to the larger form, a property called self-similarity. As the fractal (Hausdorff) dimension increases between one and two (left to right in the figure), the tree sprouts new branches more and more vigorously. The organic, treelike fractals shown here bear a striking resemblance to many physiological structures. (From West and Goldberger, 1987.)

increases with decreasing temperature T. The magnetic susceptibility, the change in the magnetization induced by a small applied field (derivative), therefore becomes singular at $T=T_c$. Thus the magnetic susceptibility is a nonanalytic function of the temperature. Renormalization group theory found its first successful application in this area of phase transitions (see, e.g. Wilson, 1979). We find that such nonanalytic functions, although present, had been thought to be exceptional in the physical sciences (Montroll and Shlesinger, 1982). However such singular behavior appears to be more the rule than the exception in social, biological and medical sciences (Sernetz, Gellén and Hoffman, 1985; Goldberger and West, 1987b; West and Salk, 1987). Before discussing these applications we need to develop some of the basic ideas regarding fractals and renormalization groups more completely.

To experimentally study these relations Underwood and Banerje undertook the numerical construction of a Koch quadratic island and a Koch triadic island. In the plot of $L(\eta)$ versus η, reproduced in Figure 2.2.6, they observed a periodicity in the experimental points which they attribute to the method of measurement. I suggest an alternate explanation based on an assumed scaling relation for the perimeter:

$$L(\eta) = \frac{1}{4} L(\eta/3) \ . \tag{2.2.9}$$

The general solution to (2.2.9) is of the form

$$L(\eta) = \frac{A(\eta)}{\eta^\alpha} \tag{2.2.10}$$

where by direct substitution we find

$$\alpha = \frac{\ln 4}{\ln 3} = d \tag{2.2.11}$$

and since

$$A(\eta) = A(\eta/3) \tag{2.2.12}$$

$A(\eta)$ is a periodic function in $\ln \eta$ with period $\ln 3$. This modulated inverse power law would clearly explain the experimental points in Figure 2.2.6. Equation (2.2.9) is an example of a renormalization group relation about which more will be said subsequently. The periodic coefficient $A(\eta)$ in (2.2.12) is often set to a constant value in which case the functional relation (2.2.9) reproduces, by iteration, the expression (2.2.3).

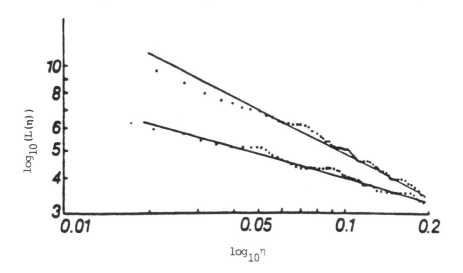

Figure 2.2.6. Experimental fractal plots for a Koch quadratic island (top curve) and a Koch triadic island (bottom curve). The apparent length $L(\eta)$ is graphed versus the measuring unit η. [From Underwood and Banerje (1986) with permission.]

Weierstrass cast the argument presented earlier on the fractal distribution of mass points into a particular mathematical form. His intent was to construct a series representation of a continuous nondifferentiable function. His function was a superposition of harmonic terms: a fundamental with a frequency ω_0 and unit amplitude, a second periodic term of frequency $b\omega_0$ with amplitude $1/a$, a third periodic term of frequency $b^2\omega_0$ with amplitude $1/a^2$, and so on (see Figure 2.2.7). The resulting function is an infinite series of periodic terms each term of which has a frequency that is a factor b larger than the succeeding term and an amplitude that is a factor of $1/a$ smaller. These parameters can be related to the Cantor set discussed earlier if we take $a = b^\mu$ with $1 < \mu < 2$. Thus, in giving a functional form to Cantor's ideas, Weierstrass was the first scientist to construct a fractal function. Note that for this concept of a fractal function, or fractal set, there is no smallest scale. For $b > 1$ in the limit of infinite N the frequency $\omega_0 b^N$ goes to infinity so there is no highest frequency contribution to the Weierstrass function. Of course if one thinks in terms of periods rather than frequencies, then the shortest period contributing to the series is zero.

Consider for a moment what is implied by the lack of a smallest scale in period, or equivalently the lack of a largest scale in frequency in the Weierstrass function depicted in the preceding figure. Imagine a continuous line on a two-dimensional Euclidean plane and suppose the line has a fractal dimension greater than unity but less than two. How would such a curve appear? At first glance the curve would seem to be a ragged line with many abrupt changes in direction (cf. Figure 2.2.8). If we now magnify a small region of the line, indicated by the box (a), we see that the enlarged region appears qualitatively the same as the original curve (cf. b). If we now magnify a small region of this new line, indicated by the box (b), we again obtain a curve qualitatively indistinguishable from the first two (cf. c). This procedure can be repeated indefinitely just as we did for the mass distribution in space. This equivalence property is called "self-similairty" and expresses the fact that the qualitative properties of the curve persist on all scales and the measure of the degree of self-similarity is precisely the fractal or Hausdorff dimension.

The Weierstrass function can be written as the Fourier series

$$F(z) = \sum_{n=0}^{\infty} \frac{1}{a^n} \cos(b^n \omega_0 z) \ , \ a, \ b > 1 \ , \tag{2.2.13}$$

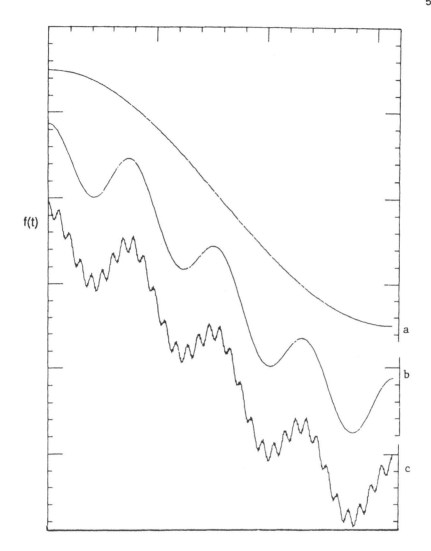

Figure 2.2.7. Here we show the harmonic terms contributing to the Weierstrass function; (a) a fundamental with frequency ω_0 and unit amplitude; (b) a second
periodic term of frequency $b\omega_0$ with amplitude $1/a$ and so on until one
obtains (c) a superposition of the first 36 terms in the Fourier series expansion of the Weierstrass function. We choose the values $a = 4$ and $b = 8$,
so that the fractal dimension is $d = 2 - 2/3 = 4/3$, close to the value used in
Figure 2.2.1.

52

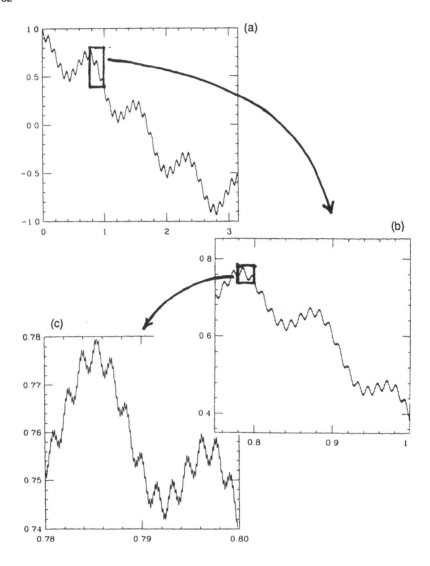

Figure 2.2.8. We reproduce here the Weierstrass curve constructed in Figure 2.2.7 in which we are superposing smaller and smaller wiggles; so that the curve looks like the irregular line on a map representing a very rugged seacoast. Inset (b) is a magnified picture of the boxed region of inset (a). We see that the curve in (b) appears qualitatively the same as the original curve. We now magnify the boxed region in (b) to obtain the curve in (c) and again obtain a curve that is qualitatively indistinguishable from the first two. This procedure can in principle be continued indefinitely because of the Hausdorff dimension of the curve.

which is the mathematical expression of the above discussion. If we now separate the $n = 0$ term from the series in (2.2.13) we can write

$$F(z) = \sum_{n=1}^{\infty} \frac{1}{a^n} \cos (b^n \omega_0 z) + \cos (\omega_0 z) \qquad (2.2.14)$$

so that shifting the series by unity we have

$$F(z) = \frac{1}{a} F(bz) + \cos (\omega_0 z) \quad . \qquad (2.2.15)$$

(In Appendix A the solution to (2.2.3) is worked out in detail.) Thus, if we drop the harmonic term on the right hand side of (2.2.15) we obtain a functional scaling relation for $F(z)$. The dominant behavior of the Weierstrass function is then expressed by the functional relation

$$F(z) = F(bz)/a \quad . \qquad (2.2.16)$$

The interpretation of this relation is that if one examines the properties of the function on the magnified scale bz what is seen is the same function observed at the smaller scale z but with an amplitude that is scaled by a. This is the self-similarity (self-affinity) discussed above, an expression of the form (2.2.16) is often called the renormalization group relation. Because we now have a mathematical expression for this self-similarity property we can predict how the function $F(z)$ varies with z. The renormalization group transformation can be solved to yield,

$$F(z) = A(z)z^{\alpha} \quad , \qquad (2.2.17)$$

where the power-law index α must be related to the two parameters in the series expansion by $\alpha = \ln a / \ln b$ just as we found earlier. Also the function $A(z)$ must be equal to $A(bz)$ so that it is periodic in the logarithm of the variable z with period $\ln b$. For example, if $A(y)$ were equal to $A(y+b)$ then $A(y)$ would be periodic in y with period b. That is the case here except that $z = \ln y$ so that the period of the function $A(z)$ is $\ln b$. The algebraic increase of $F(z)$ with z is a consequence of the scaling property of the function with z.

Mandelbrot's concept of a fractal liberates our ideas of geometric forms from the tyranny of straight lines, flat planes and regular solids and extends them into the realm of the irregular, disjoint and singular. As rich as this notion is we require one additional extension into the arena of fluctuations and probability, since it is usually in terms of averages that physiological data sets are understood. If we now interpret $F(z)$ as a random function, then in analogy with the Weierstrass function, we assume that the probability density satisfies a scaling relation. Thus the scaling property that is present in the variable $F(z)$ for the usual Weierstrass function is transferred to the probability distribution for a stochastic (random) function. This transfer implies that if the process $F(z)$ is a random variable with a properly scaled probability density then the two stochastic functions $F(bz)$ and $b^{1/\alpha}F(z)$ have the same distribution (Montroll and West, 1987). This scaling relation establishes that the irregularities of the stochastic process are generated at each scale in a *statistically identical* manner. Note that for $\alpha = 2$ this is the well known scaling property of Brownian motion with the square root of the "time" z. Thus the self-affinity that arises in the statistical context implies that the curve (the graph of the stochastic function $F(z)$ versus z) is statistically equivalent at all scales rather than being geometrically equivalent (West, 1985; Mandelbrot, 1977, 1982).

The algebraic increase of $F(z)$ with z is a consequence of the scaling property of the function with z. The scaling (2.2.17) in itself does not guarantee that $F(z)$ is a fractal function, but Berry and Lewis (1980) have studied very similar functions and concluded that they are fractal. Consider the function

$$X(z) = \sum_{n=-\infty}^{\infty} \frac{1}{a^n} \left[1 - e^{ib^n \omega_0 z} \right] e^{i\phi_n} \qquad (2.2.18)$$

where the phase ϕ_n is arbitrary. This function was first examined by Lévy and later used by Mandelbrott (1977). The fractal dimension d of the curve generated by the real part of (2.2.18) with $\phi_n = 0$ is given by 2-d = α so that

$$d = 2 - \ln a / \ln b \qquad (2.2.19)$$

which for the parameters $a = 4$ and $b = 3$, is $d = 4/3$. Maudlin and Williams (1986) examined the formal properties of such functions and concluded that for $b > 1$ and $0 < a \le b$ the dimension is in the interval $[2 - \alpha - C/\ln b, 2 - \alpha]$ where C is a positive constant and b is sufficiently large.

The set of phases $\{\phi_n\}$ may be chosen deterministically as we did above, or randomly as we do now. If ϕ_n is a random variable uniformly distributed on the interval $(0, 2\pi)$, then each choice of the set of values $\{\phi_n\}$ constitutes a member of an ensemble for the stochastic function $X(z)$. If the phases are also independent and $b \to 1^+$, then

$X(z)$ is a Gaussian random function. The condition $1 < d < 2$ is required to ensure the convergence of the sum (2.2.18).

Consider the increments of $X(z)$:

$$\Delta X(z,Z) = X(z+Z) - X(z)$$

$$= \sum_{n=-\infty}^{\infty} b^{-n(2-d)} \left[e^{ib^n \omega_0 z} - e^{ib^n \omega_0(z+Z)} \right] e^{i\phi_n} \qquad (2.2.20)$$

and assume that the ϕ_n are independent random variables uniformly distributed on the interval $(0, 2\pi)$. The mean square increment is

$$C(Z) = \left\langle |\Delta X(z,Z)|^2 \right\rangle_\phi$$

$$= \sum_{n=-\infty}^{\infty} b^{-n(4-2d)} \, 2\left[1 - \cos(b^n \, \omega_0 Z) \right] \qquad (2.2.21)$$

where the ϕ subscript on the brackets denotes an average over an ensemble of realizations of the ϕ_n-fluctuations. The right hand side of (2.2.21) is independent of z, i.e., it depends only on the difference Z, so that $\Delta X(z,Z)$ is a homogeneous (also called stationary when z is the time) random process.

Note that (2.2.21) has the same form as the real part of the extended Weierstrass function (2.2.18) when $\phi_n = 0$. If we shift the summation index in (2.2.21) by unity we obtain the scaling relation

$$C(bZ) = b^{2(2-d)} \, C(Z) \qquad (2.2.22)$$

which is of the same form as (2.2.16). Thus we see that the correlations on the extended Weierstrass function, like the function itself, is self-affine. Here again the solution to the RG relation (2.2.22) is a modulated power law.

The usual Weierstrass function was shown to increase algebraically in z with the power-law index α given by the ratio of logarithms. Therefore if either a or b is less than unity (but not both) then the sign of α will change, that is to say that the dominant behavior of $F(z)$ will be an *inverse* power-law ($1/z^\alpha$) with $\alpha = \ln a \,/\, \ln(1/b)$. The preceding interpretation of the self-similarity of a process represented by such a function remains intact if we replace the notion of going to successively smaller scales to one of going to successively larger scales. Thus an inverse power-law reflects a self-similarity under contraction whereas a power-law denotes self-similarity under magnification.

2.3   Self-Similar Physiological Structures

How do the apparently abstract notions of self-similar scaling, renormalization group theory and fractal dimensionality relate to the architecture of the lung? The classical model of bronchial diameter scaling, as we saw, predicts an exponential decay in diameter measurements (Weibel and Gomez, 1962). However the data indicate marked divergence of the observed anatomy from the predicted exponential scaling of the average diameter of the bronchial tubes beyond the tenth generation. These early arguments assume the existence of a simple characteristic scale governing the decrease in bronchial dimensions across generations. If, however, the lung is a fractal structure, no characteristic smallest scale will be present. Instead there should be a distribution of scales contributing to the variability in diameter at each generation. Based on the preceding arguments, the subsequent dominant variation of the average bronchial diameter with generation number would then be an inverse power law, not an exponential (West et al, 1986; West, 1987).

Recall that the arguments leading to the exponential form of the dependence of the average diameter of the bronchial tube with generation number z neglect the variability in the linear scales at each generation and use only average values for the tube lengths and diameters. The fractal assumption, on the other hand, focuses on this neglected variability and consequently the observed deviation of the average diameter from a simple exponential dependence on z results from the distribution in fluctuations in the linear dimensions with generation. If we interpret the Weierstrass function $F(z)$ as the diameter of the bronchial tree, then the series has two distinct contributions. One is the singular behavior of the inverse power law, which is the dependence of the average bronchial diameter on generation number and the other is an analytic, short-scale variation of the measured diameter which is averaged out in the data. The parameter b is a measure of the interval between scales that contribute to the variation in the diameter and the parameter a denotes the importance of that scale relative to its adjacent scales. In the case of the lung, in addition to the single scale assumed in the traditional models, the fractal model assumes that no single scale is dominant, but instead there is an infinite sequence of scales each a factor of b smaller than its neighbor that contribute to the structure. Each such factor b^n is weighted by a coefficient $1/a^n$. This is exactly analogous to the weighting of different frequencies in the Weierstrass function given above.

Let us now be more formal in our strategy for incorporating the variability of the diameters at each generation into the discussion. In the classical argument the average diameter is written as

$$d(z,\gamma) = d_0 e^{-\gamma z} \qquad (2.3.1)$$

where we have changed notation to explicitly account for the scale parameter $\gamma(\equiv ln(1/q) > 0)$ in the contracting process of the bronchial tree. In (2.3.1) there is a single value for γ, but in the bronchial tree there are a number of such scales present at each generation. The fluctuations in $d(z,\gamma)$ could then be characterized by a distribution of the γ's, i.e., $P(\gamma)d\gamma$ is the probability that a particular scale is present in the measured diameter. The average diameter of an airway at the zth generation is then

$$<d(z)> = \int_0^\infty d(z,\gamma) P(\gamma) d\gamma . \qquad (2.3.2)$$

If the branching process is sharply peaked at only a single scale, $\bar{\gamma}$ say, then $P(\gamma) = \delta(\gamma - \bar{\gamma})$ and (2.3.2) reduces to (2.3.1). However, we know from the data in Figure 2.1.3 that the measured average diameter $<d(z)>$ is not of the exponential form (2.3.1).

Rather than prescribing a particular functional form to the probability density West et al. (1986) formulated an argument based on a scaling of the parameter γ. Consider a distribution $P(\gamma)$ having a finite central moment, say a mean value $\bar{\gamma}$. Now, following Montroll and Shlesinger (1982), we apply a scaling mechanism such that $P(\gamma)$ has a new mean value $\bar{\gamma}/b$:

$$P(\gamma/\bar{\alpha}) \rightarrow P(b\gamma/\bar{\alpha}) \qquad (2.3.3)$$

and we assume this occurs with relative frequency $1/a$. We apply the scaling again so that the scaled mean is again scaled and the new mean is γ/b^2 and occurs with a relative frequency $1/a^2$. This amplification process is repeated over and over again and eventually generates the unnormalized distribution

$$P(\xi) = P(\xi) + \frac{1}{a} P(b\xi) + \frac{1}{a^2} P(b^2\xi) + ... \qquad (2.3.4)$$

where we introduce the dimensionless variable $\xi = \gamma/\bar{\gamma}$. Since the original distribution $P(\xi)$ is normalized to unity we obtain the normalization integral from the series (2.3.4)

58

$$\int_0^\infty P(\xi)d\xi = 1 + \frac{1}{ab} + \frac{1}{a^2b^2} + \cdots$$

$$= N(ab) \tag{2.3.5}$$

where $N(ab)$ is the normalization constant. We use the distribution (2.3.4) to evaluate the observed average diameter, denoted by an overbar, and obtain

$$\overline{d(z)} = N(ab)\left\{ <d(z)> + \frac{1}{a}<d(z/b)> + \frac{1}{a^2}\left\langle d(z/b^2) \right\rangle + \cdots \right\} \tag{2.3.6}$$

normalized to the value in (2.3.5). This series can be written in the more compact form

$$\overline{d(z)} = \frac{1}{a}\overline{d(z/b)} + N(ab)<d(z)> \tag{2.3.7}$$

as the number of terms in the series becomes infinite. The normalization constant $N(ab)$ is finite for $ab > 1$ and in fact

$$N(ab) = 1 - \frac{1}{ab} \tag{2.3.8}$$

for an infinite series.

We again note the RG relation (2.3.7) that results from this argument. Here again we restrict our attention to the dominant behavior of the solution to this RG relation. If we separate the contributions to $\overline{d(z)}$, into that due to singularities, denoted by $\overline{d_s(z)}$, and that which is analytic, denoted by $\overline{d_a(z)}$, then the singular part satisfies the functional equation

$$\overline{d_s(z)} = \frac{1}{a}\overline{d_s(z/b)} \ . \tag{2.3.9}$$

The solution to (2.3.9) we know to be

$$\overline{d_s(z)} = A(z)/z^\alpha \tag{2.3.10}$$

where by direct substitution we find

$$\alpha = ln\ a/ln\ b \tag{2.3.11}$$

and

$$A(z) = A(z/b) = \sum_{n=-\infty}^{\infty} A_n\ e^{2\pi in\ ln\ z/ln\ b} \tag{2.3.12}$$

Thus we see that the average diameter is an inverse power law in the generation index modulated by the slowly oscillating function $A(z)$ just as is observed in the data (cf. Figure 2.3.1). In point of fact we find that the present model provides an excellent fit to the lung data in four distinct species: dogs, rats, hamsters and humans. The quality of this fit shown in Figure 2.3.2 strongly suggests that the RG relation for $F(z)$ captures a fundamental property of the structure of the lung that is distinct from traditional scaling. Furthermore, the data shows the same type of scaling for bronchial tube lengths and consequently volume.

Using (2.3.10) in the expression for the average diameter of the airway (2.3.7), we obtain

$$\overline{d(z)} = \frac{A(z)}{z^{\alpha}} + B(z) \qquad (2.3.13)$$

where $B(z)$ is an analytic function. In West et al. (1986) we present the analytic form for the function $A(z)$ and $B(z)$ obtained for a particular distribution of the γ parameter values.

On a structural level the notion of self-similarity can also be applied to other complex physiological networks. The vascular system, like the bronchial tree is a ramifying network of tubes with multiple scales sizes. To describe this network Cohn (1954) introduced the notion of an "equivalent bifurcation system." The equivalent bifurcation systems were examined to determine the set of rules under which an idealized bifurcating system would most completely fill space. The analogy was based on the assumption that the branchings of the arterial system should be guided by some general morphogenetic laws enabling blood to be supplied to the various parts of the body in some optimally efficient manner. The branching rule in the mathematical system is then to be interpreted in the physiological context. This was among the first physiological applications of the self-similarity idea, predating the formal definition of fractals.

Many other fractal-like structures in physiology are also readily identified by their multiple levels of self-similar branching or foldings - for example, the bile duct system, the urinary collecting tubes in the kidney, the convoluted surface of the brain, the lining of the bowel, neural networks, and the placenta (Goldberger and West, 1987). The fractal nature of the heart is particularly striking. The cardiac surface is traversed and penetrated by a bifurcating system of coronary arteries and veins. Within its chambers,

60

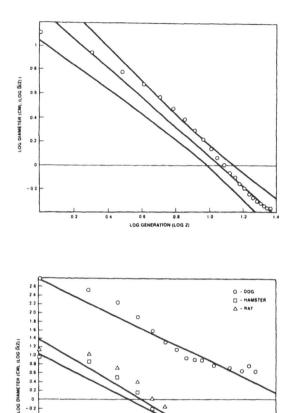

Figure 2.3.1. We plot the data of Weibel and Gomez on log-log graph paper and see that the dominant character of the functional dependence of the average bronchial diameter on generation number is indeed an inverse power law rather than an exponential. A power-law relationship between two variables appears linear when the relationship is expressed in terms of the logarithms of the variables. Thus on log-log graph paper the relationship yields a straight line (A). In addition to this inverse power-law dependence of the average diameter on z there appears to be a periodic variation of the data about this power-law behavior. This harmonic variation is not restricted to the data sets of humans but also appears in data obtained for dogs, rats and hamsters derived from Raabe and his colleagues. The harmonic variation is at least as pronounced in these latter species as it is in humans (B). (From West et al., 1985.)

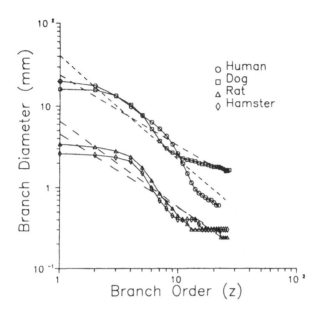

Figure 2.3.2. The variation in diameter of the bronchial airways is depicted as a function of generation numbers for rat, hamsters, and dogs. The modulated inverse power law observed in the data of Raabe et al. (1976) is readily captured by the function $F(z) = [A_0 + A_1 \cos(2\pi ln\ z/ln\ b)]/z^\mu$ (from Nelson, West and Goldberger, 1990).

branching strands of connective tissue, called chordae tendineae, anchor the mitral and tricuspal valves, and the electrical impulse is conducted by a fractal neural network, the His-Purkinje system, embedded within the muscle.

Until now we have restricted our discussion to a static context, one describing the relevance of power-law scaling and fractal dimensionality to anatomy. Such physiologic structures are only static in that they are the "fossil remnant" of a morphogenetic process. It would seem reasonable therefore to suspect that morphogenesis itself could also be described as a fractal process, but one which is time dependent. From the viewpoint of morphogenesis, the new scaling mechanisms have interesting implications regarding the development of complex but stable structures using a minimal code. One of the many challenges for future research will be unraveling the molecular and cellular mechanism whereby such scaling information is encoded and processed.

The morphogenesis of the lung has recently been modeled by Nelson and Manchester (1988) using computer simulation of growth as defined by fractal algorithms. Variations in the limits imposed by simple constraints generate structures that are in good agreement, in two dimensions, with actual structural data. In Figure 2.3.3 is depicted the computer simulation and a two-dimensional projection of an actual lung. The value in such simulations is in part related to the fact that one can test developmental and morphogenic hypothesis with varying boundary conditions including genetic effects. We have examined the fluctuation-tolerance of the growth process of the lung and found that its fractal nature does in fact have a great deal of survival potential (West, 1988). In particular it can be shown that fractal structures are much more error-tolerant than those produced by classical scaling. Such error tolerance is important in all aspects of biology, including the origins of life itself (Dyson, 1985).

The success of the fractal model of the lung suggests that nature may prefer fractal structures to those generated by more traditional scaling. We suggest that the reason as to why this is the case may be related to the tolerance that fractal structures (processes) seem to possess over and above those of classical structures (processes). Said differently, fractal processes are more adaptive to internal changes and to changes in the environment than are classical ones. Let us construct a simple quantitative model of error response to illustrate the difference between the classical and fractal models.

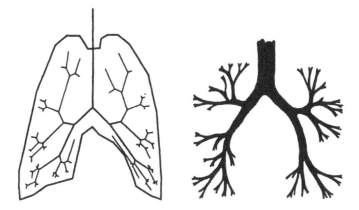

Figure 2.3.3.   A computer simulation of a fractal lung is depicted in which the boundary
condition influence the morphogenesis. The boundary was derived from a
chest radiograph. The model data are in good agreement with actual
structural data (from Nelson and Manchester, 1988 with permission).

64

Consider the theoretical average diameter of the bronchial airway given by classical scaling $d(z) = d(0) e^{-\gamma z}$. Assume that the scaling parameter γ is made up of two pieces: a constant γ_0 and a random part ξ that can arise from random changes in the environment during morphogenesis or from errors in the code generating the structure of the lung. Thus, regardless of whether the errors are produced internally or externally, the average diameter of an airway is given by

$$<d(z)>_\xi = d(0) e^{-\gamma_0 z} <e^{-\xi z}>_\xi \qquad (2.3.14)$$

where $<\cdot>_\xi$ denotes an average over an ensemble of realizations of the ξ-fluctuations. To evaluate this average we must specify the statistics of the ξ-ensemble. For convenience we assume ξ to be a zero-centered, Gaussian random variable

$$P(\xi) = \frac{1}{\sqrt{2\pi\sigma^2}} e^{-\xi^2/2\sigma^2} \qquad (2.3.15)$$

where $P(\xi) d\xi$ is the probability that the random variable lies in the interval $(\xi, \xi + d\xi)$. The first two moments of ξ are

$$<\xi>_\xi = \int_{-\infty}^{\infty} \xi P(\xi) d\xi = 0 \ , \qquad (2.3.16)$$

$$<\xi^2>_\xi = \int_{-\infty}^{\infty} \xi^2 P(\xi) d\xi = \sigma^2 \ . \qquad (2.3.17)$$

Thus, the average in (2.3.14) can be evaluated using (2.3.15) to obtain

$$<e^{-\xi z}>_\xi = \int_{-\infty}^{\infty} e^{-\xi z} P(\xi) d\xi$$

$$= \int_{-\infty}^{\infty} e^{-(\xi + \sigma^2 z)^2} \frac{d\xi}{\sqrt{2\pi\sigma^2}} e^{\sigma^2 z^2/2}$$

$$= e^{\sigma^2 z^2/2} \qquad (2.3.18)$$

so that

$$<d(z)>_\xi = <d(z)>_0 e^{\sigma^2 z^2/2} \ , \qquad (2.3.19)$$

and the error grows as $e^{\sigma^2 z^2/2}$. The assumed statistics for ξ have no significance except that it provides a specific functional form for the error that can be used to compare the classical and fractal models.

In the fractal model of the lung we assume that the power-law index consists of two pieces: a constant piece α_0 and a random piece ξ. Here again we average over the ξ-fluctuations

$$<d(z)>_\xi = \frac{A(z)}{z^{\alpha_0}}\ e^{\sigma^2(\ln z)^2/2} \qquad (2.3.20)$$

Again using (2.3.15) to evaluate the ξ-average we obtain

$$<d(z)>_\xi = <d(z)>_0\ e^{\sigma^2(\ln z)^2/2} \qquad (2.3.21)$$

so the error in the fractal model grows as $\exp[\sigma^2(\ln z)^2/2]$.

We define the error generated in the average diameter in either model as

$$\varepsilon(z) = \frac{<d(z)>_\xi}{<d(z)>_0}\ . \qquad (2.3.22)$$

In Figure 2.3.4 we graph $\varepsilon(z)$ for both the classical and fractal models. We see that the classical model propagates error in an exponential way, so that by the 12th and 13th generation, the predicted size of the airway with and without errors differs by a factor of five. An organism with this sensitivity to error (or to fluctuations in the environment during morphogenesis) would not survive over many generations of the species.

On the other hand we see that the fractal model is essentially unresponsive to error: it is very tolerant to the variability in the physiological environment. This error tolerance can be traced back to the broad band nature of the distribution in scale sizes of a fractal object. This distribution ascribes many scales to each generation in the bronchial tree, therefore any scale introduced by an error is already present, or nearly so, in the original system. Thus the fractal model *preadapts* the mammalian lung to certain genetic errors and variations in the growth environment.

In addition to morphogenesis, it seems reasonable to hypothesize that multiple other complex physiological processes would require the use of fractal concepts for their complete description. What would a time-dependent fractal process look like in a physiological context? Perhaps the most accessible way to introduce this notion is to examine a time series, which is a traditional way of assembling biomedical data sets. In this approach we examine how self-similarity can make itself manifest from one time interval to the next.

66

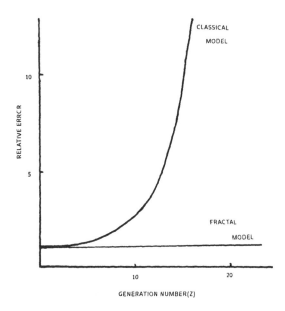

Figure 2.3.4. The error between the model prediction and that prediction with a noisy parameter is shown for the classical scaling model and the fractal model (from West, 1988).

2.4   Fractal Time Series

The usual method for analyzing biomedical time series data is to determine the harmonic content of the time trace (Basar, 1980). For an ordered set of frequencies one finds an ordered set of constants (mode amplitude), the mean square value of a given mode amplitude being the energy contained in the time series at a particular frequency. This procedure is often referred to as a spectral decomposition of the time series because it extracts from the data set (time trace) the spectrum of frequencies contributing to the process of interest. The set of moduli of the mode amplitudes determine the spectral strength of the time trace at the contributing frequencies, but the set of phases determine the detailed shape of the time trace. Thus for a prescribed spectrum the time series can represent a coherent time pulse or a random function of time and most things in-between. It is apparent that since both of these time series can have the same harmonic content it is the distribution of phases that is the central issue in determining the shape of the time trace. In the output of physiological systems both types of time series are obtained; coherent pulses as well as apparently random time traces, see e.g. Figure 2.4.1.

The dramatic difference between the extremes of coherent signals and random noise is a manifestation of the different dynamics present in the processes generating the phase relations between the different spectral components. The time series for the pulse is reminiscent of the QRS-complex observed in an electrocardiogram. The QRS is the representation of the depolarization of the myocardial cells. The erratic time series with its apparently random phase, on the other hand, is reminiscent of heart rate variability in an active healthy subject or the EEG of an alert mammalian brain (cf. Chapter 4).

If we interpret the usual series for the fractal function $F(z)$, given by (2.2.13) to be the spectral decomposition of a time series where the previously discrete z is interpreted as the continuous time t, then it represents a dynamic process that does not have a time derivative. For a continuous time series the energy content is determined by means of the autocorrelation function which measures how long the influence of a given variation in a times series persists. The autocorrelation function is obtained by multiplying $F(t)$ by a displaced copy of itself $F(t+\tau)$ and integrating t over a long time interval T and dividing by T in the limit T becomes infinite:

68

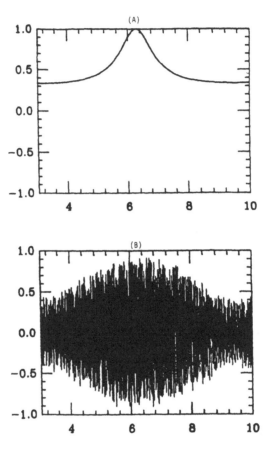

Figure 2.4.1. We select frequencies that are integer multiples of a fundamental frequency ω_0 and the amplitudes decrease according to a scaling rule such that the nth amplitude is a factor $1/a$ smaller than the $(n-1)$st. Then the spectrum consists of the harmonics of ω_0 with the nth harmonic having a spectral strength $1/a^{2n}$. The shape of a time trace having this spectrum is quite variable. If we choose all the phases to have a constant value, zero say, curve (A), then the time trace is given by a single pulse of height $a/(a-1)$. If we choose the phases to be random variables, uniformly distributed on the interval $(0, 2\pi)$, curve (B), the resulting time trace appears to be a random function of time.

$$C(\tau) = \lim_{T \to \infty} \frac{1}{T} \int_{-T/2}^{T/2} F(t) F(t+\tau) \, dt \quad . \tag{2.4.1}$$

The interesting aspect of the extended Weierstrass function is that its autocorrelation function also has the form of the extended Weierstrass function, but with different parameters (Berry and Lewis, 1980). We can now use the properties of this function that we developed earlier to interpret the correlation function. The first is that since $F(t)$ has a modulated power law as its dominant time behavior [see (2.2.17)], then so too does the auto-correlation function of the time series, but with twice the power-law index:

$$C(\tau) = \lim_{T \to \infty} \frac{1}{T} \int_{-T/2}^{T/2} dt \sum_{n=0}^{\infty} \sum_{n'=0}^{\infty} \frac{1}{a^{n+n'}} \cos b^n \omega_0 t \, \cos b^{n'} \omega_0 (t+\tau) \quad . \tag{2.4.2}$$

Using the trigonometric identity for the product of cosines and the integral relation

$$\frac{1}{2\pi} \int_{-\pi}^{\pi} d\theta \cos m\theta \, \cos m'\theta = \delta_{m,m'} \tag{2.4.3}$$

we obtain

$$C(\tau) = \sum_{n=0}^{\infty} \frac{1}{a^{2n}} \cos(b^n \omega_0 \tau) \tag{2.4.4}$$

so that following the analysis in Appendix A gives the dominant behavior for the correlation function

$$C(\tau) = A(\tau) \tau^{2\alpha} \quad , \tag{2.4.5}$$

where $\alpha = \ln a / \ln b$ and $A(\tau)$ is again a slowly varying periodic function in $\ln \tau$. The energy spectral density of the time series is given by the Fourier Transform of the correlation function,

$$S(\omega) = \int_{-\infty}^{\infty} d\tau \, e^{i\omega\tau} C(\tau) \quad . \tag{2.4.6}$$

Due to the slow variation of $A(\tau)$ with time the asymptotic spectrum is estimated using a Tauberian Theorem (see e.g. Wiener, 1963) to be

$$S(\omega) \approx 1/\omega^{2\alpha+1} \tag{2.4.7}$$

for small ω, which is an inverse power law in the frequency.

The above argument indicates that a fractal time series should be associated with a power spectrum in which the higher the frequency component, the lower its power. Furthermore, if the spectrum is represented by an inverse power law, then a plot of log (frequency) versus log (power) should yield a straight line graph of slope $-(2\alpha+1)$. Since the frequency output of physiological systems can be a determined using Fourier analysis, this scaling hypothesis can be directly tested.

Let us now return to our example of the cardiac depolarization pulse. Normally, each heartbeat is initiated by a stimulus from pacemaker cells in the sinus node in the right atrium. The activation wave then spreads through the atria to the AV junction. Following activation of the AV junction, the cardiac impulse spreads to the ventricular myocardium through a ramifying network, the His-Purkinje system. This branching structure of the His-Purkinje conduction system is strongly reminiscent of the bronchial fractal we discussed earlier. In both structures, one sees a self-similar tree with finely-scaled details on a "microscopic" level. The spread of this depolarization wave is represented on the body surface by the QRS-complex of the electrocardiogram. Spectral analysis of the QRS waveform (time trace) reveals a broadband frequency spectrum with a long tail corresponding to an inverse power law in frequency. To explain this inverse power-law spectrum we (Goldberger et al., 1985b) have conjectured that the repetitive branchings of the His-Purkinje system represent a fractal set in which each generation of the self-similar segmenting tree imposes greater detail onto the system. At each fork in this network, see Figure 2.4.2, the cardiac impulse will activate a new pulse along each conduction branch, thus yielding two pulses for one. In this manner, a single pulse entering the proximal point of the His-Purkinje network with N distal branches, will generate N pulses at the interface of the conduction network and myocardium. In a fractal network, the arrival times of these pulses at the myocardium will not be uniform. The effect of the finely branching fractal network will be to subtly *decorrelate* the individual pulses that superpose to form the QRS-complex (Goldberger et al., 1985b).

As we have discussed, a fractal network is one that cannot be expressed in terms of a single scale, so that one cannot express the overall decorrelation rate of impulses by a single time scale. Instead one finds a distribution of decorrelation rates in the time trace in direct correspondence to the distribution of branch lengths in the conduction network. These rates are based on an infinite series in which each term corresponds to

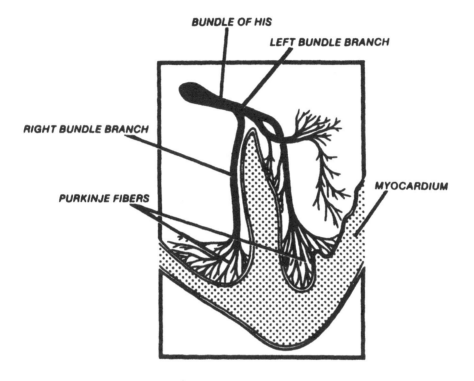

Figure 2.4.2. The ventricular conduction system (His-Purkinje) appears to be a fractal-
           like structure demonstrating repetitive branching on progressively smaller
           scales.

higher and higher mean decorrelation rates in direct analogy with the series expansion for the Weierstrass function. Each term therefore represents the effect of superposing finer and finer scales onto the fractal structure of the conduction system. Each new "layer" of structure renormalizes the distribution of mean decorrelation rates. This renormalization procedure eventually leads to a transition in the distribution of decorrelation rates to a power-law form in the region of high decorrelation rates. The spectrum of the time trace of the voltage-time pulses resulting from this fractal decorrelation cascade of N pulses will also show inverse power-law behavior.

We have argued that a voltage pulse emanating from the pacemaker model region of the heart becomes shattered into a large number of equal amplitude pulses. Each pulse travels a different path length to reach the myocardium and there superimposes to form the classical QRS pulse. The distribution in path lengths resulting from the fractal nature of the branches gives rise to a distribution of decorrelation times τ_c among the individual spikes impinging on the myocardium. The unknown distribution $p(\tau_c)$ can be obtained using an argument parallel to that presented for the mammalian lung.

We denote the correlation function constructed from the time series for the QRS complex by $c(t)$ and assume it has a maximum correlation time τ_c, e.g., it has the exponential form e^{-t/τ_c}. We use the argument leading to (2.3.6) by considering a sequence of shorter correlation times each with a relative frequency $1/a$. Let $c(t)$ be amplified such that its correlative time is τ_c/b. Again in the second stage of amplification, which we assume occurs with relative frequency $1/a^2$, the basic correlation time τ_c becomes τ_c/b^2. The new correlation function $C(t)$ containing continuing levels of amplification is

$$C(t) = \left[1 - \frac{1}{a}\right] \left\{ c(t) + \frac{b}{a} c(bt) + \frac{b^2}{a^2} c(b^3 t) + \cdots \right\} \qquad (2.4.8)$$

so that

$$C(t) = \frac{b}{a} C(bt) + \frac{a-1}{a} c(t) \ . \qquad (2.4.9)$$

The solution to (2.4.9) as $t \to \infty$ is given by

$$C(t) = A(t) t^{\alpha-1} \ , \qquad (2.4.10)$$

where as before $\alpha = \ln a / \ln b$ and again $A(t)$ is a periodic function in $\ln t$ with fundamental period *ln b*.

The power spectrum $S(\omega)$ for the *QRS* pulse is

$$S(\omega) = 2 \int_0^\infty dt \, A(t) \, t^{\alpha-1} \cos \omega t \quad . \tag{2.4.11}$$

Again, if $A(t)$ is slowly varying in time or is constant, the integral (2.4.11) can be evaluated using a Tauberian Theorem to be

$$S(\omega) \sim \frac{1}{\omega^\alpha} \quad . \tag{2.4.12}$$

In a general study the exponent α can depend on other parameters such as temperature and pressure. Thus according to this argument the *QRS* waveform should have an inverse power-law spectrum.

The actual data fits this model quite well (see Figure 2.4.3). This example, therefore, supports another connection between nonlinear structures, represented by a fractal His-Purkinje system, and nonlinear function, reflected in the inverse power-law pulse (Goldberger and West, 1987b). Thus, just as nature selects static anatomical structures with no fundamental length scale, he/she selects a structure for the His-Purkinje conduction system so as to have no fundamental time scale. Presumably the error-tolerance of the fractal structure is as strong an influence on the latter as it is on the former. The next and related question is whether self-similar scaling mechanisms also regulate higher order physiological phenomena which represent the interaction of *multiple* processes.

To take a specific example suggested earlier, does self-similar scaling contribute to the regulation of a complex process such as heart rate variability? One can obtain a crude measure of heart-rate variations by feeling one's own pulse. With a casual observation, the pulse rate may feel quite even, but on closer inspection it clearly is not a strictly regular event. For example, an increase in pulse rate is noted with inspiration (and a decrease with expiration). These oscillations are called *phasic* or *respiratory* arrhythmia. Other more subtle variations in heart rate have been detailed by means of spectral decomposition through which oscillations at other frequencies have been correlated with physiologic temperature and blood pressure control mechanisms.

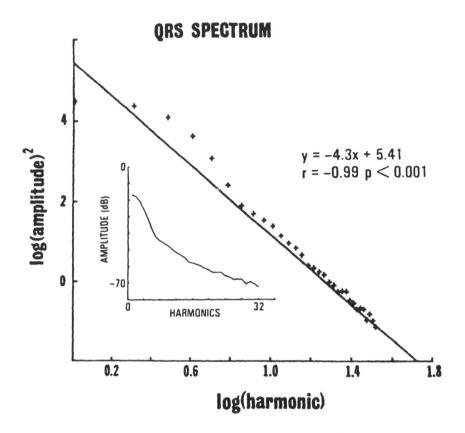

Figure 2.4.3. The normal ventricular deploration (QRS) waveform (mean data of 21 healthy men) shows a broadband distribution with a long, high-frequency tail. The straight line is the linear regression to an inverse power-law spectrum [$S(\omega) \sim 1/\omega^{\alpha}$] with a fundamental frequency of 7.81 Hz. (Goldberger et al., 1985 with permission.)

However, such periodic changes account for only a part of the overall fluctuations in heart rate. To measure this variability more comprehensively, we should record the heart beat over a long period of observation when the subject is going about his or her daily activities, unencumbered by the restrictions of a controlled environment. This kind of analysis was performed recently by Kobayashi and Musha (1982). They performed power spectral analyses of heart rate time series data obtained by ambulatory healthy subjects wearing a portable ECG device. Remarkably, the spectra for the heart rates in the healthy subjects were very similar and of particular interest to the present analysis, they showed an inverse power-law pattern with a superimposed peak corresponding to the respiratory frequency. Thus, heart rate variability shows an inverse power law suggesting the type of scaling behavior noted in a variety of other physiological contexts.

In the case of the *QRS*-complex such power-law scaling could be related to the fractal geometry of the His-Purkinje system. What is the "mechanism" for self-similar scaling in the regulation of heart rate variability? Fluctuations in heart rate are regulated by multiple control processes including neurohumoral regulation (sympathetic and parasympathetic stimulation), and local electrochemical factors. One strategy for ascertaining the contribution of such factors would be to selectively block their effects, for example by giving the drug propranolol to eliminate sympathetic effects or atropine to block parasympathetic effects. Such experiments have been very helpful in assessing the directional effect of various modulators of heart rate and estimating their quantitative contributions. However, this type of experimental methodology does not address the basis of the inverse power-law spectrum observed when the entire system is functioning normally. When we pose the question: "What is the mechanism of such inverse power-law spectra?" we are not searching for a mechanism in the conventional sense. Traditionally in physiology, the term mechanism applies to the linear interaction of two or more (linear or nonlinear) elements which *causes* something to happen. Receptor-ligand binding, enzyme substrate interactions, and reflex-arcs are all examples of traditional physiological mechanisms. The "mechanism" responsible for inverse power-law behavior in physiological systems, however, is probably not a result of a linear interactive cause-effect chain, but more likely relates to the kinds of complex scaling interactions we have been discussing. The inverse power-law spectrum can be viewed as the resultant of possibly many processes interacting over a myriad of interdependent scales.

One image that suggests itself is that of a feedback system which induces a response on time scaled a factor of b smaller than the input time. When this scaled response is fed back as part of the input, it generates a second scaled response on a time scale that is again a factor b smaller than the response of the preceding time scale. This is an application of Weiner's concept of Cybernetics (Wiener, 1968) that is of particular physiological importance. It is a control feedback system whose self-similar scaling property enhances the stability of the system response. In the conventional control system the spectrum of the control mechanism is usually a smooth function centered on a frequency ω_0 and tapering rapidly to zero over some restricted interval of frequency in the neighborhood of $\omega = \omega_0$. For the system envisioned here, the feedback control yields a total spectrum which is an inverse power law in frequency due to the lack of a highest characteristic frequency. The stability of the power-law system is greater than that of the normal feedback system since if any one element of feedback in a self-similar cascade is lost it would not significantly affect the overall system response characteristics. This is true because the series of response times is *lacunary*, i.e., it has gaps, rather than being continuous. Therefore one or a few additional gaps in the series would not change the control properties of the feedback. This is similar to the fluctuation-tolerance we observed in the fractal structure of the lung (West, 1987;1988).

This self-similar feedback hypothesis, of course, does not specifically answer the more basic question of how the multiple scales are actually generated. What the hypothesis suggests is that this type of general scaling mechanism is at play. Elucidating the basis of this generic scaling from the molecular level on up is one of the major challenges for ''nonlinear'' fractal physiology.

2.5   Fractal Summary

In this chapter we have discussed the fact that there is not one, but three contexts in which one finds fractals; geometrical, statistical, and dynamical. A geometrical fractal has to do with the static structure of an object, and stretches our notions of geometry beyond that of a point, line and plane and the accompanying concepts of smoothness and continuity, into the realm of the irregular and discontinuous. The classical geometry of Euclid is concerned with regular forms in integer dimensions. However, as we saw, anatomical shapes are perversely non-Euclidean as is apparent by looking at, say, the mammalian lung and His-Purkinje conduction system of the heart. Fractal geometry is concerned with irregular forms in these non-integer dimensions.

Statistical fractals share a number of characteristics with geometrical fractals. We saw, for example, that the latter possessed a structural self-similarity, so that as one magnifies a given region of such a structure then more and more structural detail is revealed. Correspondingly in a statistical fractal, one finds a statistical self-similarity. In a fractal stochastic process, not only does the process itself display a kind of self-similarity, but so too does the distribution function characterized the statistics of the process. For example if $X(t)$ is a random function of time, if it is fractal, then for constant $\beta > 1$ and $\alpha > 1$ we have $X(t) = \beta^{-\alpha} X(\beta t)$, i.e., a given realization $X(t)$ is identical with one that has been stretched in time (βt) and scaled in amplitude ($\beta^{-\alpha}$) where α is related to the fractal dimension. In the case of the lung the statistics were not time dependent since the scales appearing there are the consequence of its asymptotic (in time) state. The fractal character of the statistics reveals itself in that case in the inverse power-law distribution function specifying the statistics of the scales contributing to the linear scales of the bronchial tubes at each generation in the lung. Recall that the inverse power law is a consequence of the statistics having no fundamental scale, just as the geometrical fractal has no fundamental spatial scale.

Finally, we recall that a dynamical fractal was used in the interpretation of the His-Purkinje conduction system as a fractal network. In this example we observed that there was no fundamental time scale (period) in the fractal process, resulting in a correlation function that increased algebraically in time. This power-law correlation function resulted in a predicted inverse power-law spectrum of the QRS-complex which was also observed.

The physiological examples considered in this chapter share the common feature of being static. Even the time dependence of the correlation function obtained from the QRS time series resulted from the static structure of the His-Purkinje conduction network rather than as a consequence of any time varying aspect of the system. In subsequent chapters we are also concerned with the dynamic aspect of physiology, including *dynamical diseases* as well as the other aspects of physiology and medicine that are intrinsically time dependent.

Appendix A. Scaling of the Weierstrass Function

The scaling property of the Weierstrass function (2.2.13) was determined in detail by Hughes et al. and we follow their argument here. The nonanalytic behavior of $F(z)$ at $z = 0$ is revealed by writing the cosine in terms of its inverse Mellin transform with respect to z:

$$\cos(b^n \omega_0 z) = \frac{1}{2\pi i} \int_{C-i\infty}^{C+i\infty} \frac{\Gamma(s)\cos(\pi s/2)}{(b^2 \omega_0 z)^s} \, ds \ , \ 0 < c = Re(s) < 1 \ . \tag{A.1}$$

The Weierstrass function can then be written as

$$
\begin{aligned}
F(z) &= \frac{1}{2\pi i} \int_{C-i\infty}^{C+i\infty} ds \ \frac{\Gamma(s)\cos(\pi s/2)}{(\omega_0 z)^s} \sum_{n=0}^{\infty} \frac{1}{(ab^s)^n} \\
&= \frac{1}{2\pi i} \int_{C-i\infty}^{C+i\infty} ds \ \frac{\Gamma(s)\cos(\pi s/2)}{(\omega_0 z)^s \left[1 - 1/ab^s\right]}
\end{aligned}
\tag{A.2}
$$

where the series has been explicitly summed. Hughes et al. (1981) noted that the integral is a meromorphic function of s, with single poles at $s = 0, -2, -4, \cdots$ due to the factor $\Gamma(s)\cos(\pi s/2)$ and at $s = -\mu + 2\pi ni/\ln b, n = 0, \pm 1, \pm 2 \cdots$ due to the zeros in the denominator, where

$$\alpha = \ln a / \ln b \ . \tag{A.3}$$

If the contour of integration is translated to $Re(s) = -\infty$ and the residues of the poles over which the contour passes are properly accounted for, they obtain

$$F(z) = z^\alpha Q(z) + \sum_{m=0}^{\infty} \frac{(-1)(\omega_0 t)^{2m}}{(2m)! \left[1 - \dfrac{b^{2m}}{a}\right]} \ , \tag{A.4}$$

where

$$Q(z) = \frac{\omega_0}{\ln b} \sum_{n=-\infty}^{\infty} \Gamma\left(-\alpha + \frac{2\pi ni}{\ln b}\right) \cos\left[\left(-\alpha + \frac{2\pi ni}{\ln b}\right)\pi/2\right] e^{-2\pi ni \frac{\ln(\omega_0 z)}{\ln b}} . \tag{A.5}$$

The analysis leading to (A.4) and (A.5) can be justified rigorously when $1/2 < \mu < 2$, and by introducing a convergence factor extended to $0 < \mu < 1/2$ as well.

Thus the Weierstrass function separates into a nonanalytic part that carries the singular behavior of the function $z^\alpha Q(z)$ since $Q(z)$ is an analytic function, and an analytic part denoted by the series in (A.4). Asymptotically the singular part of $F(z)$ dominates and one obtains the behavior given by (2.2.15).

3. DYNAMICS IN FRACTAL DIMENSIONS

Up until now we have focused our attention primarily on the relevance of the new scaling ideas to structure and function in physiology. We now redirect that attention to the dynamics intrinsic to a large number of biomedical systems. In the present chapter we attempt to present some of the formal ideas of nonlinear dynamic systems theory, and to relate these ideas to those presented in the previous chapters. Of obvious additional interest are the potential medical implications of these concepts. If, for example, normal function of a variety, and perhaps all, physiological systems is characterized by inverse power-law distributions, then a reasonable hypothesis is that at least some disease states will be associated with a loss of this normal scaling.

How will these scaling pathologies be evidenced? At present, only very preliminary answers can be given to this important question. Mackey and Milton (1987) and earlier Mackey and Glass (1977) defined a dynamic disease as one that occurs in an intact physiological control system operating in a range of control parameters that leads to abnormal dynamics. This is consistent with the definition used by Goldberger and West (1987a, 1985a). The signature of the abnormality is a change in the qualitative dynamics of some observable as one or more parameters are changed. The power spectrum of the process is one such measure of the normal operating state. A number of disease processes appear to be characterized by a narrowing of the frequency spectrum with a relative decrease in higher frequency components. We have observed a similar loss of ''spectral reserve'' in cardiac interbeat interval spectra following atropine administration to normal subjects (Goldberger and West, 1987b). Thus, it appears that interference with the autonomic nervous system leads to a loss of spectral reserve.

A related feature of the frequency spectra of perturbed physiological systems is that not only is overall power reduced, but spectral energy may eventually become confined to a few *discrete* frequency bands. The discrete (narrowband) type of frequency spectrum contrasts with the broadband inverse power-law spectra seen under normal conditions. The shift from a broadband to a narrowband spectrum dramatically alters the behavior of the system. Instead of observing physiological variability, one will begin to see highly periodic behavior. The medical literature abounds with examples of such ''pathological (usually low frequency) periodicities.'' For example, low-frequency, periodic fluctuations in heart rate and respiration may be a prominent feature in patients with severe congestive heart failure (Goldberger, Findley, Blackburn and Mandell, 1987; Goldberger et al., 1986) as well as in the fetal distress syndrome (Modanlon and Freeman, 1982). This cyclic behavior of respiration in very ill cardiac patients has actually been known for several centuries, and is referred to as the *Cheyne-Stokes breathing* (see Figure 3.0.1). It is also observed in obese persons, and after neural brainstem lesions. The detection of a loss of spectral reserve and the onset of pathological periodicities in both adults and infants at risk for sudden death promises to provide a new approach to cardiovascular monitoring.

Furthermore, similar techniques may provide novel ways of monitoring other systems. For example an inverse power-law spectrum characterizes the apparently erratic daily fluctuations in counts of neutrophils (a type of blood cell) in healthy subjects. In contrast, periodic (predictable) fluctuations in neutrophil counts have already been detected in certain cases of chronic leukemia (Goldberger, Kabalten and Bhargava, 1986). These oscillations have periods of between 30 and 70 days depending on the patient. This periodic behavior along with the fluctuations have been modeled using single deterministic time delay equations (see e.g. Mackey and Milton, 1987). Such models will be discussed more fully subsequently. Spectral analysis of fluctuations in blood counts may provide a useful means of identifying preleukemic states and also perhaps of following patients' responses to chemotherapy. Finally, a loss of physiological variability in a variety of systems appears to be characteristic of the aging process in different organ systems (Waddington, Mac Collock and Sambrooks, 1979; Mandell, 1988; Goldberg, West and Bhargava, 1985a).

Neurological disorders, including epilepsy and movement disorders, have also been modeled as dynamic diseases in which the role of bifurcation has been examined, see Rapp (1986) for a review. Rapp, Latta and Mees (1988) point out that in 1932 Gjessing published the first in a series of papers establishing the correlation between intermittent catatonia (periodic catatonia schizophrenia) and rhythmic changes in the basal metabolic rate. These variations and the schizophrenic symptoms persisted unless treated by thyroxin (Donziger and Elmergreen, 1954). More biomedical examples will be discussed subsequently after we have developed the fundamental concepts of nonlinear dynamics.

In all these areas of medical research, there is a common physiological theme. Complexity is the salient feature shared by all the systems we have discussed - a feature that is attracting more and more attention in physical systems as well (Goldberger and

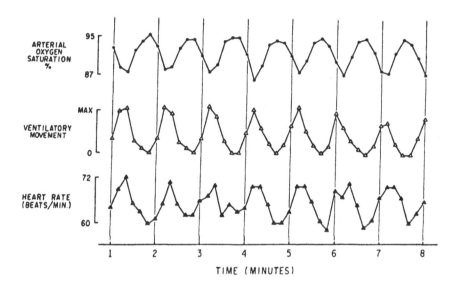

Figure 3.0.1. The low frequency periodic fluctuations in the heart rate are compared with two measure of respiration in very ill cardiac patients. The phenomenon is referred to as *Cheyne-Stokes breathing*.

West, 1987a). Until today, scientists have assumed that understanding such systems in different contexts, or even understanding various physiological systems in the same organism, would require completely different models. The most exciting prospect for the new dynamics is that is may provide a unifying theme to many investigations which up to now have been considered unrelated.

3.1 Nonlinear Bio-Oscillator

In the physical sciences the dynamics of a system are determined by the equations describing how the physical observables change in time. These equations are obtained by means of some general principle, such as the conservation of energy and/or the conversation of momentum, applied to the system of interest. The appropriate conservation law follows from a symmetry of the system which determines a rule by which the system evolves. If a set of circumstances is specified by an N-component vector $X = (X_1, X_2, .., X_N)$ then in order to predict the future state of the system from its present configuration, we must specify a rule for the systems' evolution. In the physical sciences the traditional strategy is to construct a set of differential equations. These equations are obtained by considering each component of the system to be a function of time, then as time changes so too do the circumstances. If in a short time interval Δt we can associate an attendant set of changes $\Delta X = (\Delta X_1, ..., \Delta X_N)$ as determined by $\Delta X = F(X, t)\Delta t$ then in the limit $\Delta t \rightarrow 0$ one would write the "equations of motion."

$$\frac{d}{dt} X(t) = F(X, t) \tag{3.1.1}$$

which is a statement about the evolution of the system in time. If at time $t = 0$ we specify the components $X(0)$, i.e., the set of circumstances characterizing the system, and if $F(X, t)$ is an analytic function of its arguments, then the evolution of the system is determined by direct integration of the equations of motion away from the initial state. This is one of the styles of thought adopted from the physical sciences into the biological and behavioral sciences (West, 1985).

The mathematicians have categorized the solutions to such equations for the simplest kinds of systems. One way to describe such systems is by means of geometric constructions in which the solution to an equation of the above form is depicted by a curve in an appropriate space. The coordinate axes necessary for such a construction are the continuum of values that the vector $X(t)$ can assume, each axis being associated with one component of the vector $\mathbf{X}$. As we saw in the Introduction, this is called a phase space. Consider a two-dimensional phase space having axes labeled by the components of the dynamical system $\mathbf{X} = (X_1, X_2)$. A point in the phase space $\mathbf{x} = (x_1, x_2)$ gives a complete characterization of the dynamical system at a point in time. As time proceeds this point traces out a curve as shown in Figure 3.1.1, starting from the initial state $[X_1(0), X_2(0)]$ and proceeding to the final state $[X_1(t), X_2(t)]$ at time t. A trajectory or orbit in phase space traces out the evolution of the dynamical system. Time is a continuous parameter which indexes each point along such a solution curve. The field of trajectories initiated from a set of initial conditions is often referred to as the flow field. If for example the flow field asymptotically ($t \to \infty$) converges to a single point in phase space, this is called a fixed point (or focus) (cf. Figure 3.1.2). If the flow field converges to a single closed curve this is called a limit cycle (cf. Figure 3.1.3). Such limit cycles appear as periodic time series for the variables of interest.

Nature abounds with rhythmic behavior that closely intertwines the physical, biological and social sciences. The spinning earth gives rise to periods of dark and light that are apparently manifest through the circadian rhythms in biology. An incomplete list of such daily rhythms is given by Luce (1971): the apparent frequency in fetal activity variations in body and skin temperature, the relative number of red and white cells in the blood along with the rate at which blood will coagulate, the production and breakdown of ATP (adenosine triphosphate), cell division in various organs, insulin secretion in the pancreas, susceptibility to bacteria and infection, allergies and pain tolerance. No attempt has been made here to distinguish between cause and effect; here we only stress the observed periodicity in each of these phenomena. The shorter periods associated with the beating of the heart and breathing, for example, are also modulated by a circadian rhythm.

There is a tendency to think of the rhythmic nature of many biological phenomena, such as the beating of the heart, breathing, circadian rhythm, etc. as arising from the dominance of one element of a biosystem over all the other elements. A logical consequence of this mode of thought is the point of view that much of the biosystem is passive, taking information from the dominant element and merely passing it along through the system to the point of utilization. This perspective is being called into question more and more by the mathematical biologists, a substantial number of which regard the rhythmic

84

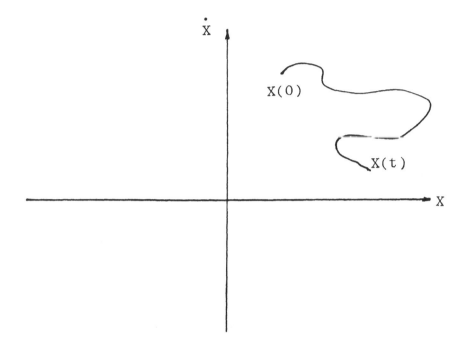

Figure 3.1.1.   The $(x, \dot{x})$ plane constitutes a two-dimensional phase space for a dynamical system. The curve is a schematic representation of the instantaneous
state of the system, starting form the initial point labeled $t = 0$. Time (not
shown) is a parameter that locates the system along the trajectory.

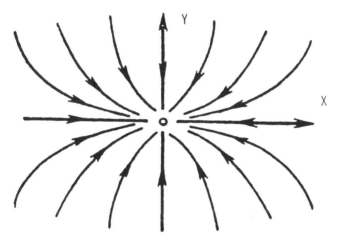

Figure 3.1.2. The collection of trajectories initiated from a set of initial conditions is called a flow field. Here the flow field in the neighborhood of a fixed point is shown. All the trajectories asymptotically converge on the single point in phase space, i.e., they reside in the basin of attraction of the focus.

86

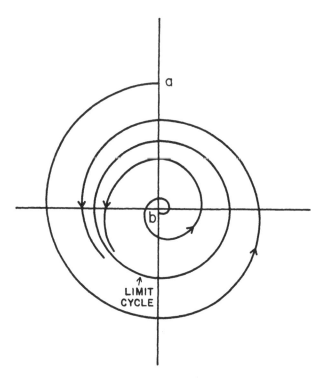

Figure 3.1.3. The two points *a* and *b* in the figure are possible initial conditions for the system. When the system can manifest limit cycle behavior the orbits approach this cycle asymptotically and lose all memory of their initial state.

nature of biological processes to be the consequence of a dynamic interactive nonlinear network, that is to say that biological systems are systemic (see e.g. Koslow, Mandell and Shlesinger, 1987). The mathematical models used to support this contention were first developed in the evolving discipline of nonlinear dynamics which is emerging as a new discipline out of physics and applied mathematics. The application of some of the techniques of nonlinear dynamics to biological oscillations is of recent origin being championed by Winfree (1977, 1984), Glass et al. (1982, 1983), West and Goldberger (1987) among others. The application of nonlinear equations to describe biorhythms, however, actually dates back to the 1929 work of van der Pol and van der Mark on the *relaxation oscillator*.

Oscillations in biological processes do not in general follow a simple harmonic variation in either space or time. The usually situation is one in which the period of oscillation is dependent on a number of unrelated factors, some intrinsic to the system but others external to it. Examples of these factors are the amplitude of the oscillation, the period at which the biological unit is being driven, the internal dissipative processes and fluctuations, to name a few. In particular, since all biological units are thermodynamically open to the environment they give up energy to their surroundings in the form of heat, i.e., they are dissipative. This regulatory mechanism helps to maintain the organism at an even temperature. Thus, if a simple harmonic oscillator is used to realistically simulate an organism undergoing oscillations, it must contain dissipation. It is well known, however, that the asymptotic trajectory of a dissipative linear oscillator is a stable fixed point in phase space. The phase space in this case consists of the oscillator displacement $X(t)$ and velocity $\dot{X}(t)$ as depicted in Figure 3.1.4. Here the amplitude of the oscillator excursions become smaller and smaller, due to dissipation, until eventually it comes to rest.

If a bio-oscillator is to remain periodic, energy must be supplied to the organism in such a way as to balance the continuous loss of energy due to dissipation. If such a balance is maintained then the phase space orbit will become a stable *limit cycle*, i.e., all orbits in the neighborhood of this orbit will merge with it asymptotically. However, simple oscillators do not have the appropriate qualitative features for describing biological systems. One of the important properties that linear oscillators lack and which is apparently ubiquitous

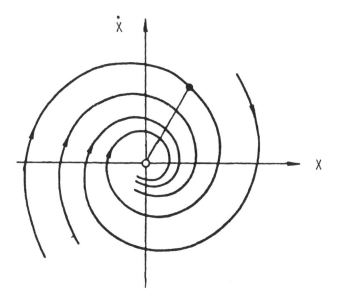

Figure 3.1.4. The trajectories of a linear harmonic oscillator with dissipation are shown in the $(x, \dot{x})$ phase space to be spirals centered on the origin. The origin $(x = 0, \dot{x} = 0)$ is the fixed point of this dynamic system.

among biological systems is that of being self-starting (see Section 3.2). Left to itself a bio-oscillator will spontaneously begin to oscillate without external excitation. One observes that the self-starting or self-regulating character of bio-oscillators depends on the intrinsic nonlinearity of the organism. Examples of systems that experimentally manifest this self-regulating behavior are aggregates of embryonic cells of chick hearts (Glass, Guevara and Perez, 1983), simian cortical neurons (Rapp, Zimmerman, Albano, Deguzman and Greenbaum, 1985) and the giant internodel cell of the fresh water algae *Nitella flexilis* (Hayashi, Nakao and Hirakawa, 1982) to name a few. The experimental data from these and other examples are discussed in Chapter 4.

A nonlinear oscillator which is "weakly" nonlinear is capable of oscillating at essentially a single frequency and can produce a signal that is very low in harmonic content. Although the output from such an oscillator system is sinusoidal at a single frequency, there are fundamental and crucial differences between such an oscillator and the classical harmonic oscillator, the latter being a conservative linear system which is lossfree. The basic difference is that the nonlinear oscillator can oscillate at one and only one frequency and at one and only one amplitude, the amplitude and frequency are dependent on one another for a given configuration of parameters. In contrast, the amplitude and frequency are independent in the classical linear oscillator, which can oscillate at any arbitrary level for a given set of parameter values. These differences are illustrated in the description of the limit cycle. The phase plane of a Hamiltonian (loss-free) oscillator is depicted in Figure 3.1.5 together with the limit cycle for an oscillator with nonlinear dissipation (cf. Figure 3.1.6). Although there are superficial resemblances between these diagrams, there are, in fact, fundamental differences between these two physical systems. While the linear conservative oscillator can be described by an infinite family of closed ellipses, as shown in Figure 3.1.5, the nonlinear oscillator approaches a *single limit cycle* as seen in Figure 3.1.6. This limit cycle is reached asymptotically whether the initial conditions correspond to an infinitesimal perturbation near the origin or to a finite perturbation far beyond the limit cycle. In either case the phase point spirals to the limit cycle, which is a stable final state. On the other hand, the conservative linear oscillator does not display this "structural stability." Any perturbation causes it to leave one ellipse and move to another where it stays, i.e.,the orbits are neutrally stable.

90

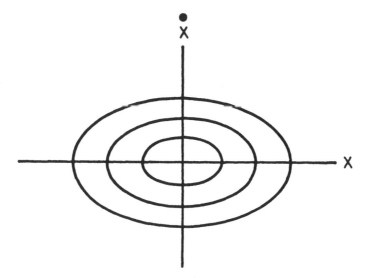

Figure 3.1.5.   The $(\dot{x}, x)$ phase space is shown for a harmonic oscillator with a few typical orbits. Each ellipse has a constant energy. As the energy of the oscillator is increased the system jumps from an ellipse of smaller diameter to
one of larger diameter.

91

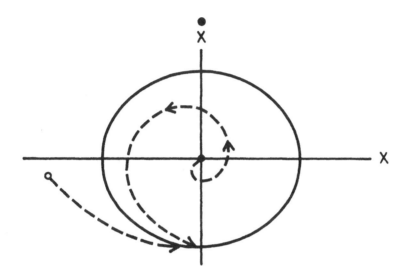

Figure 3.1.6. A single limit cycle is depicted (solid curve). The dashed curves corresponds to transient trajectories that asymptotically approach the limit cycle.

In linear systems the term equilibrium is usually applied in connection with conservative forces, with the point of equilibrium corresponding to the balancing of all forces with the system staying at rest. The stability of such an equilibrium state is then defined by the behavior of the system when it is subject to a small perturbation i.e., a small displacement away from the equilibrium state in phase space. Roughly speaking, the terms stability and instability indicate that after the perturbation is applied the system returns to the equilibrium state (stable) or that it continues to move away from it (unstable) or that it does not move at all (neutral stability). One of the first places where these ideas can be found in a biological context is in Lotka's 1925 book on mathematical biology.

To set these ideas in a familiar context we adopt the nomenclature that a bio-oscillator is one that is self-excitatory; regardless of the initial state of the system it will approach a stable limit cycle providing that no pathologies arise. This idea of an active system was originally proposed in 1928 by van der Pol and van der Mark, using a nonlinear dynamic equation of the form

$$\frac{d^2V(t)}{dt^2} - \left[\varepsilon^2 - V^2(t) \right] \frac{dV(t)}{dt} + \omega_0^2 V(t) = 0 \ , \tag{3.1.2}$$

where $V(t)$ is the voltage, ω_0 is the natural frequency, and ε is an adjustable parameter. In a linear oscillator of frequency ω_0 the coefficient of the first order time derivative determines the stability property of the system. If this coefficient, say λ, is positive then the system is asymptotically stable, i.e., there is a damping $e^{-\lambda t}$ so that the oscillator approaches the fixed point $V = 0$ in phase space. If the coefficient λ is negative the solution diverges to infinity as time increases without limit $(e^{|\lambda| t})$. Of course this latter behavior must terminate eventually since time divergences do not exist in physical or biological systems for all time, at worst stability is lost; usually other mechanisms come into play to saturate the secular growth. In the nonlinear system (3.1.2) the "coefficient" of the "dissipative" term changes sign depending on whether $V^2(t)$ is greater than or less than ε^2. This property of (3.1.2) leads to a limit cycle behavior of the trajectory in the $(\dot{v}, v)$-phase space for the system (cf. Figure 3.1.6). The above authors envisioned the application of this limit cycle paradigm to "explain" a great many phenomena such as:

"the aeolian harp, a pneumatic hammer, the scratching noise of a knife on a plate, the waving of a flag in the wind, the humming noise sometimes made by a water tap, the squeaking of a door, a neon tube, the periodic recurrence of epidemics and of economic crisis, the periodic density of an even number of species of animals living together and the one species serving as food for the other, the sleeping of flowers, the periodic recurrence of showers behind a depression, the shivering from cold, menstruation and, finally, the beating of the heart.''

Although the van der Pal oscillator given by (3.1.2) does not have the broad range of application envisioned by van der Pal and van der Mark (1928,1929), their comments reveal that they understood that these many and varied phenomena are dominated by nonlinear mechanisms. In this sense their remarks are prophetic.

We now take up the last example in the above quote in some detail.

(a)   The cardiac oscillator*

Under physiologic conditions, the normal pacemaker of the heart is the sino-atrial (SA) node – a collection of cells with spontaneous automaticity located in the right atrium. The impulse from the SA node spreads through the atrial muscle (triggering atrial contraction). According to the traditional viewpoint, the depolarization wave then spreads through the atrioventricular (AV) node (junction) and down the His-Purkinje system into the ventricles. The fundamental premise in this model is that the AV node functions during normal sinus rhythm as a passive conduit for impulses originating in the SA node, and that the intrinsic automaticity of the AV node is suppressed during sinus rhythm. This view assumes that the AV node does not actively generate impulses or otherwise influence the SA node (Vassalle, 1977).

The alternate viewpoint of van der Pol and van der Mark, and the one adopted here, is that the AV node functions as an active oscillator and not simply as a passive resistive element in the cardiac electrical network (Guevara and Glass, 1982; Katholi, Urtholer, Macy and James, 1977; Ikeda, 1982; Goldberger and West, 1987b). An active role of the AV node is supported by the clinical observation that, under certain conditions, the sinus and AV nodes may become functionally disassociated so that independent atrial (P) and ventricular (QRS) waves are seen on the electrocardiogram (AV disassociation). Further, if the SA node is pharmacologically suppressed, or ablated, then the AV node assumes an active pacemaker role. The intrinsic rate of this AV nodal pacemaker is about two-thirds of that of the SA node in dogs (Katholi et al., 1977) and possibly in man.

In contrast to the traditional passive conduit theory of the AV node, nonlinear analysis suggests that the SA and AV nodes may function in an active and interactive

*This section borrows heavily from West et al. (1985).

way, with the faster firing SA node appearing to entrain the AV node (West, Goldberger, Rovner and Bhargava, 1985). This entrainment should be bi-directional, not uni-directional, with the SA node both influencing and being influenced by the AV node. Previous nonlinear models (Guevara and Glass, 1982; Katholi et al., 1977; Ikeda, 1982) of the supraventricular cardiac conduction system did not explicitly incorporate this bi-directional type of interaction.

To simulate bi-directional SA-AV node interactions, we here adapt a computer model of two coupled nonlinear oscillators first developed by Gollub, Brunner and Danby (1978), to describe trajectory divergence of coupled relaxation oscillators. The circuit includes two tunnel diodes-electronic components (cf. Figure 3.1.7) with the same type of nonlinear voltage-current relationships found in physiological pacemakers with hysteresis properties (cf. Figure 3.1.8). The dynamics of the coupled system can be better visualized if we consider the two branches of the circuit separately. Consider a single oscillator in isolation, which for an appropriate choice of V_0 and resistance R_1, an instability drives the circuit into oscillations in which the loop indicted in Figure 3.1.8 is continually traversed in a period of order L_1/R_1. The diode current I_{D_1} (in this case $I_{D_1} = I_1$) then has the form of a rising exponential for low voltage (V_L) and descending exponential for high voltage (V_H). The voltage switches between these high and low valves when I_{D_1} attains the threshold values I_L or I_H. The parameter values (L_j/R_j) of each of the isolated oscillators are set to take into account the intrinsic difference in rate between the two pacemakers (AV/SA = 2/3).

The two oscillators are coupled together by the conductances $G_c \equiv 1/R_c$ and $G = 1/R$. The state of the circuit is defined by a point in the four-dimensional phase space with coordinate axes $(I_{D1}, I_{D2}, V_{D1}, V_{D2})$. The coupling results in a voltage drop $(V_{D1} - V_{D2})$ across R_c, producing a current through each diode dependent on this voltage drop, and can result in induced switching of one oscillator by the other. The time rates of change in the current through the two diode branches of the circuit are determined by Kirchhoff's laws:

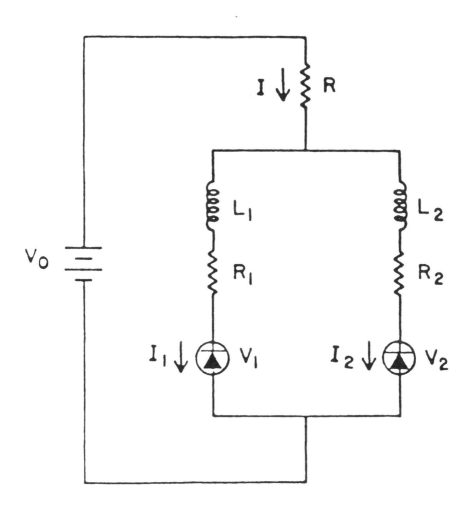

Figure 3.1.7. Analog circuit described by Equations (3.1.3) and (3.1.4) with tunnel diodes, resistors and inductors. The overall voltage is provided by the batter V_0 with the total current I. (From West et al., 1985.)

96

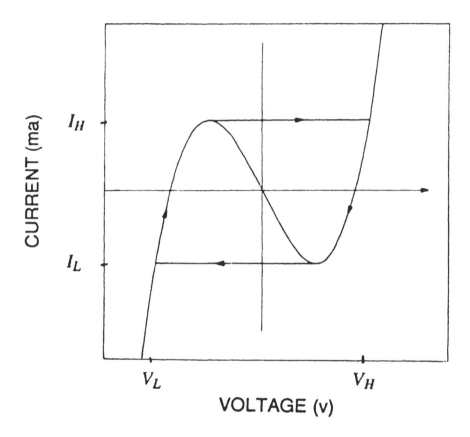

Figure 3.1.8. A typical voltage response curve across a diode is shown. The highest current is I_H, the lowest current is I_L, the highest voltage is V_H and the lowest voltage is V_L. The arrows indicate how the diode operation jumps discontinuously to V_H at constant I_H, and to V_L at constant I_L.

$$L_1 \frac{dI_1(t)}{dt} + (R + R_1)I_1(t) + R_2 I_2(t) = V_0 - V_{D1} \qquad (3.1.3)$$

$$L_2 \frac{dI_2(t)}{dt} + (R + R_2)I_2(t) + R_1 I_1(t) = V_0 - V_{D2} \qquad (3.1.4)$$

and

$$I_{D1} = I_1 + I_c \qquad (3.1.5)$$

$$I_{D2} = I_2 - I_c \qquad (3.1.6)$$

$$I_c = (V_{D2} - V_{D1})G_c \quad . \qquad (3.1.7)$$

Gollub, Romer and Socolar (1980) approximated the current-voltage characteristics of the diode (cf. Figure 3.1.8) to be rectangular, so that $V_{D1} = V_L$ (a constant) as the current increases from I_L to I_H and $V_{D1} = V_H$ (a constant) as the current decreases from I_H back to I_L. However, they include in the V_L and V_H the voltage drop across the diode caused by the coupling current I_c:

$$V_L = |I_c R_D| \; , \quad V_H = 0.45V - |I_c R_D| \; , \qquad (3.1.8)$$

where the diode resistance R_D is taken to be 5 Ω.

The equations (3.1.3) and (3.1.4) constitute a coupled feedback system through the I_2-dependence of the $\dot{I}_1$ equation and the I_1-dependence of the $\dot{I}_2$-equation . The two oscillators are linearly coupled by means of the resistors R and R_c, and each one is driven by the voltage difference between the source and that dropped across the diode introducing the anharmonic effect of the current-voltage response curve (cf. Figure 3.1.8). Because the tunnel diodes are hysteretic (nonlinear) devices, as the current in one of them increases, the voltage across it remains nearly the same (V_L) until the current reaches I_H, at which time the voltage suddenly switches to V_H ($>V_L$). At this point the current begins to decrease again with little or no change in the voltage until the current reaches the value I_L, at which point the voltage switches back to V_L. The cycle then repeats itself. The cycling of the coupled system is depicted in Figure 3.1.9 which shows that the sharply angled regions of the uncoupled hysteresis loops have been smoothed out by means of the couping. Here we use the model of Gollub et al. (1980) in which the transition between V_L and V_H on the upper branch and between V_H and V_L on

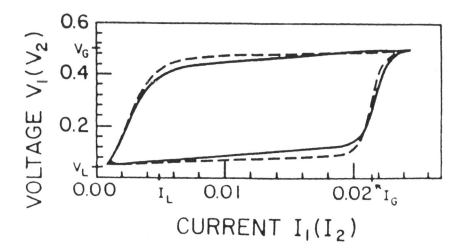

Figure 3.1.9. The hysteresis cycle of operation across the diode, is depicted. The sharp changes in voltage shown in Figure 3.1.8 are here smoothed out by the coupling between diodes. (From West et al., 1985.)

the lower branch of the hysteresis loop is instantaneous, because of its simplicity. West et al. (1985) have generalized this model to mimic the smooth change from one branch of the hysteresis curve to the other that is observed in physiological oscillators by replacing the above discontinuity with a hyperbolic tangent function along with a voltage which linearly increases in magnitude with time at the transition point I_H and I_L.

We have included two distinct types of coupling in our dynamic equations. The first is through the resistor R since the voltage applied to one oscillator now depends on the current being drawn by the other one. The second coupling is through the cross resistor R_c which directly joins the two diodes. In this latter case the current through the diode is not the same as that drawn by the inductor in the oscillator, but is modified by the current through the cross couping resistor, i.e., it depends on the relative values of $V_1(t)$ and $V_2(t)$.

Let us consider first the dynamics of the two coupled oscillators with only the R-couping present. This is accomplished by setting $G_c = 0$ ($R_c = \infty$) in (3.1.7) resulting in $I_c = 0$. The dynamics of the coupled system can be depicted by the orbits in the reduced phase space (I_1, I_2) for a certain set of system parameter values. Basically we observe that all four of the dynamic variables, the two voltage $V_1(t)$ and $V_2(t)$, and the two currents $I_1(t)$ and $I_2(t)$, are strictly periodic with period T for all applied voltages V_0 at which oscillations in fact occur. A periodic solution to the dynamic equations (3.1.3) and (3.1.4) is a closed curve in the reduced phase space as shown in Figure 3.1.10. Here, for two periods in one oscillator we have three in the other so that the coupled frequencies are in the ratio of three to two. A closed orbit with $2m$ turns along one direction and of $2n$ turns in the orthogonal direction indicate a phase locking between the two diodes such that one diode undergoes n cycles and the other m cycles in a constant time interval T for the coupled system. Figure 3.1.11 also shows the time trace of the voltage across diodes 1 and 2 for this case. We observe the 3:2 ratio of oscillator frequencies over a broad range of values of V_0.

For an externally applied voltage less than 0.225V the frequency ratio of the two oscillators becomes phase locked (one-to-one coupling) at a frequency that is lower than the intrinsic frequency of the SA mode oscillator, but faster than that of the AV junction oscillator. In Figure 3.1.12 the output of both oscillators in the coupled system is depicted, with parameter values such that the uncoupled frequencies are in the ratio of three

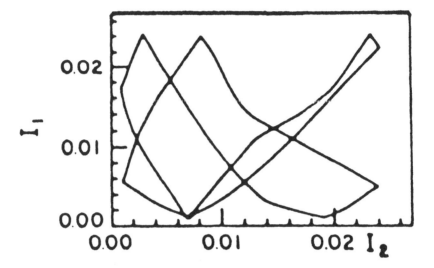

Figure 3.1.10.   The current in diode 1 is graphed as a function of the current through
diode 2. We see that the trajectory forms a closed figure indicating the
existence of a limit cycle   ($R = 3.2$ Ω, $V_0 = 0.32$ V, $R_1 = 1.3$ Ω, L_1
$= 2.772 \mu H$, $R_2 = 1.4 \Omega$, $L_2 = 3.732 \mu H$). (From West et al., 1985.)

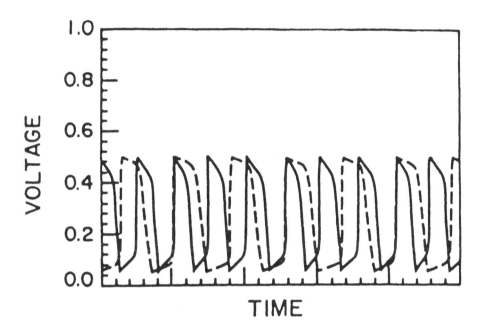

Figure 3.1.11.   Voltage pulses are shown as a function of time (dimensionless units) for
                 SA (solid line) and AV (dashed line) oscillators with parameter values
                 given in Figure 3.1.10. Note that there are two AV pulses for three SA
                 pulses, i.e., 3:2 phase locking. (From West et al., 1985.)

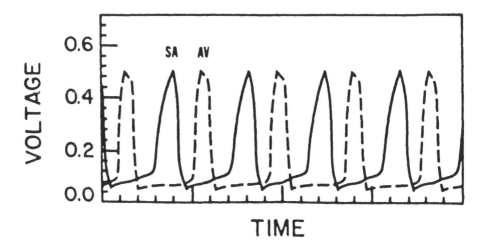

Figure 3.1.12.   Voltage pulses are shown as a function of time (dimensionless units) for
SA (solid line) and AV (dashed line) oscillators with voltage given by
$V_0 = 0.182V$ and the remaining parameters the same as in Figure
3.1.10. The limit cycle in this case is 1:1 phase locked. (From West et
al., 1985.)

to two. In the coupled system, the SA and AV oscillators are clearly one-to-one phase locked due to their dynamic interaction.

To simulate the effects of driving the right atrium at increasing rates with an external pacemaker (an experiment done on dogs in the laboratory) (Katholi et al., 1977), an external voltage of variable frequency was applied to the SA node oscillator branch of the circuit. Externally "pacing" the SA oscillator results in the appearance of a 3:2 Wenckebach-type periodicity over a initial range of driving frequencies. Furthermore, when the system is driven beyond a critical point, a 2:1 "block" occurs with only every other SA pulse being followed by an AV pulse (cf. Figure 3.1.13).

While the type of equivalent circuit model given here is not unique, it does lend support to a nonlinear concept of cardiac conduction. In particular, the model is consistent with the viewpoint that normal sinus rhythm involves a bi-directional interaction (one-to-one phase locking) between coupled nonlinear oscillators that have intrinsic frequencies in the ratio of about 3:2. Furthermore, the dynamics suggest that AV Wenckebach and 2:1 block, which have traditionally been considered purely as conduction disorders, may at least, under some conditions, relate to alterations in the nonlinear coupling of these two active oscillators. Apparent changes in conduction, therefore, may under certain circumstances be epiphenomenal. The present model demonstrates that abrupt changes (bifurcations) in the phase relation between the two oscillators occur when the intrinsically faster pacemaker is driven at progressively higher rates. In the present model, over a critical range of frequencies, a distinctive type of periodicity is observed such that the interval between the SA and AV oscillators becomes progressively longer until one SA pulse is not followed by an AV pulse. This cycle then repeats itself, analogous to AV Wenckebach periodicity which is characterized by progressive prolongation of the PR interval until a P-wave is not followed by a QRS-complex. These AV Wenckebach cycles, which may be seen under a variety of pathological conditions, are also a feature of normal electrophysiological dynamics and can be induced by driving the atria with an electronic pacemaker (Josephson and Seides, 1979).

The findings of both phase-locking and bifurcation-like behavior are particularly noteworthy in this two oscillator model because they emerge without any special assumptions regarding conduction time between oscillators, refractoriness of either oscillator to repetitive stimulation or the differential effect of one oscillators on the other.

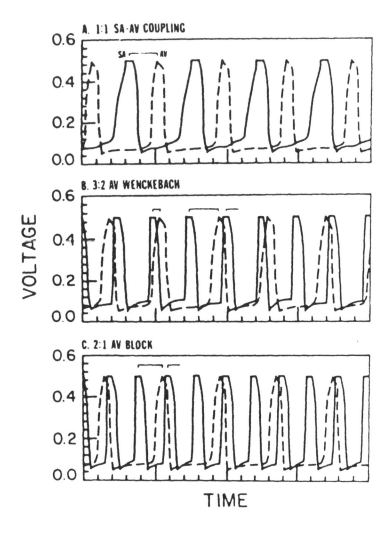

Figure 3.1.13.   Voltage pulses with the same parameter values as in Figure 3.1.10; (A) 1:1 phase locking persists when the SA node is driven by an external voltage pulse train with pulse width 0.5 dimensionless time units and period 4.0. (B) Driver period is reduced to 2.0 with emergence of 3:2 Wenckebach periodicity. (C) Driver period reduced to 1.5, resulting in a 2:1 AV block. Closed brackets denote SA pulse associated with AV response. Open brackets denote SA pulse without AV response ("non-conducted beat"). (From West et al., 1985.)

The observed dynamics support the contention that the AV junction may be more than a passive conduit for impulses generated by the sinus node, is also suggested by Guevara and Glass (1982). The present model is consistent with the alternative interpretation that normal sinus rhythm corresponds to one-to-one phase locking (entrainment) of two or more active oscillators, and does not require complete suppression of the slower pacemaker by the faster one, as do the passive conduit models. It should be emphasized, however, that when two active pacemakers become one-to-one phase locked, the intrinsically slower one may be mistaken as a passive element because of its temporal relation to the intrinsically faster one. Furthermore, the model is of interest because it demonstrates marked qualitative changes in system dynamics, characteristics of AV Wenckebach and 2:1 AV block, occurring when a single parameter (driving frequency) is varied over some critical range of values.

Up to this point we have been using the traditional concepts of a limit cycle to discuss one kind of dynamic process, ie., the beating of the heart and the occurrence of certain cardiac pathologies. We could extend this discussion to model various of the other biorhythms mentioned earlier, but that is not our purpose here. Rather we are interested in exploring certain of the modern concepts arising in nonlinear dynamics and investigating how they may be applied in a biomedical context. Let us therefore proceed and develop those ideas that will eventually be of value in understanding both erratic ECG EEG time series. It is apparent that the classical limit cycle is too well ordered to be of much assistance in that regard, so let us turn to an attractor that is a bit strange.

(b) Strange attractors (deterministic randomness)

The appellation ''strange attractor'' was given to those attractors on which, unlike the system discussed in the preceding subsection, the dynamics give rise to trajectories that are aperiodic. This means that a deterministic equation of motion gives rise to a trajectory whose corresponding time series nowhere repeats itself over time; it is chaotic. The term ''chaotic'' refers to the dynamics of the attractor, whereas ''strangeness'' refers to the topology of the attractor. Juxtaposing the words deterministic and chaotic, the former indicating the property of determinability (predictability) and the latter that of randomness (unpredictability), usually draws an audience. The expectation of people is that they will be entertained by learning how the paradox is resolved. The resolution of the apparent conflict between the traditional and modern view of dynamic systems theory as presented in classical mechanics, so eloquently stated by Laplace and Poincaré, respectively, in the Introduction, is that chaos is not inconsistent with the traditional notion of solving deterministic equations of evolution. As Ford (1987) states:

" . . . Determinism means that Newtonian orbits exist and are unique, but since existence-uniqueness theorems are generally nonconstructive, they assert nothing about the character of the Newtonian orbits they define. Specifically, they do not preclude a Newtonian orbit from passing every computable test for randomness of being humanly indistinguishable from a realization of a truly random process. Thus, popular opinion to the contrary notwithstanding, there is absolutely no contradiction in the term "deterministically random." Indeed, it is quite reasonable to suggest that the most general definition of chaos should read: chaos means deterministically random . . "

From the point of view of classical statistical mechanics the idea of randomness has traditionally been associated with the weak interaction of an observable with the rest of the universe. Take for example the steady beat of the heart, it would have been argued that a heart beat is periodic and regular. The beat-to-beat variability that is in fact observed (cf. Chapter 2) would be associated with changing external conditions such as the state of exercise, the electro-chemical environment of the heart, and so on. The traditional view requires there to be many (an infinite number) degrees of freedom that are not directly observed, but whose presence is manifest through fluctuations. More recently it has been learned that in a nonlinear system with even a few degrees of freedom chaotic motion can be observed (see e.g. West, 1985).

What we present in this subsection are some of the recent results obtained in nonlinear dynamics that lead to chaos. First we briefly review the classical work of Lorenz (1963) on a deterministic continuous dissipative system with three variables. The phase space orbit for the solution to the Lorenz system is on an attractor, but of a kind on which the solution is aperiodic and therefore the attractor is *strange*. We discuss this family of aperiodic solutions and discover that chaos lurks in a phase space of dimension three. Rössler (1978) points out that if oscillation is *the* typical behavior of low-dimensional dynamical systems, then chaos, in the same way, characterizes three-dimensional continuous systems.

Thus, if nonlinearities are ubiquitous then so to must be chaos. This led Ford to speculate on the existence of a generalized uncertainty principle based on the notion that the fundamental measures of physics are actually chaotic. The perfect clocks and meter sticks of Newton are replaced with "weakly interacting chaotic substitutes" so that the act of measurement itself introduces a small and uncontrollable error into the quantity being measured. Unlike the law of error conceived by Gauss, which is based on linearity and the principle of superposition of independent events, the postulated errors arising from nonlinearities cannot be reduced by increasing the accuracy of one's measurements. The error (noise) is generated by the intrinsic chaos associated with physical being.

In his unique style Ford (1987) summarizes those speculations in the following way:

> "Although much, perhaps most, of man's impressive knowledge of the physical world is based on the analytic solutions of dynamical systems which are integrable, such systems are, metaphorically speaking, as rare as integers on the real line. Of course, each integrable system is "surrounded" . . . by various other systems amenable to treatment by perturbation theory. But even in their totality, these systems form only an extremely small subset of the dynamical whole. If we depart this small but precious oasis of analytically solvable, integrable or nearly integrable systems, we enter upon a vast desert wasteland of undifferentiated nonintegrability. Therein the trackless waste, we find the nomads: systems abandoned because they failed a qualifying test for integrability; systems exiled for exhibiting such complex behavior they were resistant to deterministic solution they were labeled intractable. Of course, we also find chaos in full residence everywhere . . . "

The modern view of randomness discussed in the Introduction can be traced back to Poincaré, but the recent avalanche of interest dates from the attempts of Lorenz to understand the short term variability of weather patterns and thereby enhance their predictability; subsequently we consider a number of biomedical examples. His approach was to represent a forced dissipative geophysical hydrodynamic flow by a set of deterministic nonlinear differential equations with a finite number of degrees of freedom. By forcing we mean that the environment provides a source of energy for the flow field, which in this case is a source of heat at the bottom of the atmosphere. The dissipation in this flow extracts energy from the temperature gradient but the forcing term puts energy back in. For the particular physical problem Lorenz was investigating, the number of degrees of freedom he was eventually able to use was three, by convention let's call them X, Y, and Z. In the now standard form these equations are

$$\frac{dX}{d\tau} = -\sigma X + \sigma Y \qquad (3.1.9)$$

$$\frac{dY}{d\tau} = -XZ + rX - Y \tag{3.1.10}$$

$$\frac{dZ}{d\tau} = XY - bZ \tag{3.1.11}$$

where σ, r and b are parameters. The solutions to this system of equations can be identified with trajectories in phase space. What is of interest here are the properties of nonperiodic bounded solutions in this three dimensional phase space. A bounded solution is one that remains within a restricted domain of phase space as time goes to infinity.

The phase space for the set of equations (3.1.9) - (3.1.11), is three-dimensional and the solution to them traces out a curve $\Gamma_t(x,y,z)$ given by the locus of values of $X(t) = [X(t), Y(t), Z(t)]$ (cf. Figure 3.1.14). We can associte a small volume $V_0(t) = X_0(t)Y_0(t)Z_0(t)$ with a perturbation of the trajectory and investigate how this volume of phase space changes with time. If the original flow is confined to a region R then the rate of change of the small volume with time $\partial V_0/\partial t$ must be balanced by the flux of volume $J(t) = V_0(t)\dot{X}(t)$ across the boundaries of R. The quantity $\dot{X}(t)$ in the flux J represents the time rate of change of the dynamical variables in the absence of the perturbations, i.e., the unperturbed flow field that can sweep the perturbation out of the region R. The balancing condition is expressed by an equation of continuity and in the physics literature is written

$$\frac{\partial}{\partial t} V_0(t) + \nabla \cdot J(t) = 0 \tag{3.1.12}$$

or substituting $J = V_0\dot{X}$ into (3.1.12) and reordering terms yields

$$\frac{1}{V_0(t)} \frac{d}{dt}V_0(t) = \partial_X \dot{X} + \partial_Y \dot{Y} + \partial_Z \dot{Z} \quad , \tag{3.1.13}$$

where d/dt $(\equiv \partial_t + \dot{x}\cdot\nabla_x)$ is the so-called *convective* or *total* derivative of the volume. Using the equations of motion (3.1.9) - (3.1.11) for the time derivatives in (3.1.13) we obtain

$$\frac{1}{V_0(t)} \frac{d}{dt}V_0(t) = -(\sigma + b + 1) \quad . \tag{3.1.14}$$

Equation (3.1.14) is interpreted to mean that as an observer moves along with an element of phase space volume $V_0(t)$ associated with the flow field, the volume will contract at a rate $b + \sigma + 1$, i.e., the solution to (3.1.14) is $V_0(t) = V_0(t=0) \exp[-(b+\sigma+1)t]$.

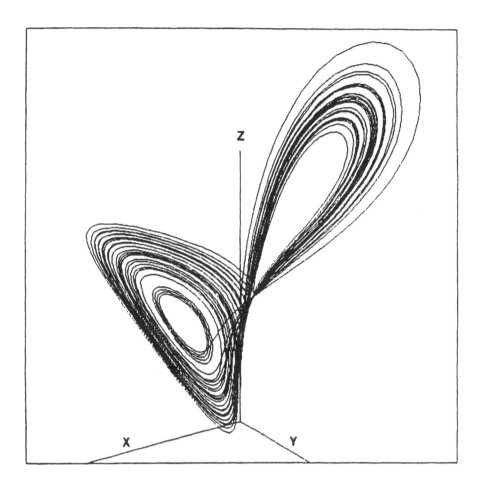

Figure 3.1.14.   The attractor solution to the Lorenz system, equations (3.1.9)-(3.1.11), is depicted in a three-dimensional phase space (X,Y,Z). The attractor is *strange* in that it has a fractal (noninteger) dimension. (From Schaffer, 1985 with permission.)

Hence the volume goes to zero as $t \rightarrow \infty$ at a rate which is independent of the solutions $X(t), Y(t)$ and $Z(t)$ and dependents only on the parameters σ and b. As pointed out by Lorenz, this does not mean that each small volume shrinks to a point in phase space; the volume may simply become flattened into a surface, one with a fractional dimension, i.e., a non-integer dimension between two and three. Consequently the total volume of the region initially enclosed by the surface R shrinks to zero at the same rate, resulting in all trajectories become asymptotically confined to a specific subspace having zero volume and a fractal dimension (Ott, 1985).

To understand the relation of this system to the kind of dynamical situation we were discussing in the preceding section we must study the behavior of the system on the limiting manifold to which all trajectories will be ultimately confined. This cannot be done analytically because of the nonintegrable nature of the equations of motion (3.1.9) - (3.1.11). Therefore, these equations are integrated numerically on a computer and the resulting solution is depicted as a curve in phase space for particular values of the parameters σ, b and r. The technical details associated with the mathematical understanding of these solutions is available in the literature, see e.g. Ott (1985) or Eckmann and Ruelle (1985) and of course the original discussion of Lorenz (1963).

In Figure 3.1.15 we display the behavior of $Y(t)$ for 3000 time units. After reaching an early peak at $t = 35$, $Y(t)$ relaxes to a relatively stable value at $t = 85$ which persists, subject to systematically amplified oscillations, until near $t \approx 1650$. Beyond this time $Y(t)$ becomes pulse-like and appears to change signs at apparently random intervals. This irregularity is not just in the spacing between maxima but also in the sign of the adjacent maxima, i.e., the irregular occurrence of a number of peaks of one sign before a peak of the opposite sign occurs.

In Figure 3.1.16a the solution manifold in the three-dimensional phase space is shown and (3.1.16b) projects the solution manifold onto the (z, y)-plane and the (x, y)-plane. The trajectory indicated is not complete, but is that segment traversed in the time interval $t = 1400$ to 1900. The points C and C' are the fixed points of the equations, i.e., the values of x, y, and z for which $\dot{X} = \dot{Y} = \dot{Z} = 0$ in (3.1.9)-(3.1.11), which for $r > 1$ yield $X = Y = \pm[b(r-1)]^{1/2}, Z = r-1$. These two views of the trajectory indicate that the erratic behavior apparent in the $Y(t)$ plot (cf. Figure 3.1.15) arises from the orbit

y(t)

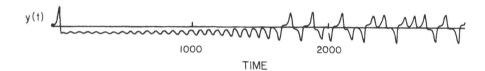

1000   2000

TIME

Figure 3.1.15.   The time history of the $Y(t)$ component of the solution to the Lorenz system of equations (3.1.9)-(3.1.11) is shown for 3×10^3 time units (from Lorenz, 1963).

112

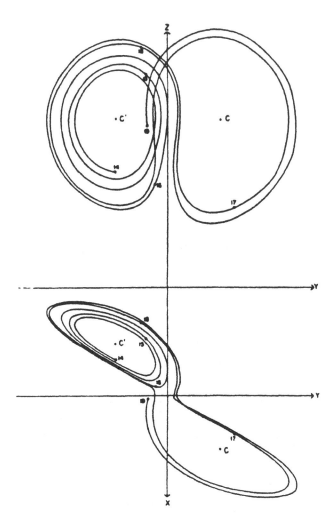

Figure 3.1.16.   Numerical solution of the convection equations. Projections on the X−Y-plane and the Y−Z-plane in phase space of the segment of the trajectory extending from iteration 1400 to iteration 1900. Numerals "14," "15," etc., denote positions at iterations 1400, 1500, etc. States of steady convection are denoted by C and C'.

spiraling around one of the fixed points C or C' for some arbitrary period and then jumping to the vicinity of the other fixed point, spiraling around that for a while and then jumping back to the other and on and on. If the number of times the orbit circled C and C' were recorded and ordered, the resulting sequence would be random. Virtually all trajectories finally end up on this highly unstable manifold.

The strange attractor depicted in Figure 3.1.14 is not the only solution to the Lorenz system of equations. This solution was obtained for the parameter values $\sigma = 10$, $b = 8/3$, $r = 28$. If the values $\sigma = 10$ and $b = 8/3$ are held fixed and r is increased from zero, a wide range of attractors and subsequent dynamic behaviors are obtained. The possible flow patterns make the transition from stable equilibria independent of initial conditions, to chaotic attractors that are sensitively dependent on initial conditions, to "chaotic transients" (Yorke and Yorke, 1979) in which, for certain initial conditions, an apparently chaotic trajectory emerges and asymptotically decays into a stable equilibria. The decay time is a sensitive function of the initial state.

Lorenz, in examining the solution to his equations, deduced that the trajectory is apparently confined to a surface. Ott (1985) commented that the apparent "surface" must have a small thickness, and it is inside this thickness that the complicated structure of the strange attractor is embedded. This is where the folding discussed in the Introduction actually occurs. If one were to pass a transverse line through this surface, the intersection of the line with the surface would be a set of dimension d with $0 \le d \le 1$. This fractional dimension indicates that the intersection of the line and surface is a Cantor set such as depicted in Figure 2.1.1. The structure of the attractor is therefore fractal, and the stretching and folding of the trajectory discussed earlier is a geometric property of the attractor.

The erratic behavior in the time series depicted in Figure 3.1.15 is also apparent in the associated power spectrum. The spectrum is the mean square value of the Fourier transform of a time series, i.e., the Fourier transform of the correlation function. Consider the solution of one component of the Lorenz system, say $X(t)$; it will have a Fourier transform over a time interval T defined by

$$\hat{X}_T(\omega) = \int_{-T/2}^{T/2} X(t)\, e^{-i\omega t}\, \frac{dt}{2\pi} \qquad (3.1.15)$$

and a power spectral density (PSD)

$$S_{xx}(\omega) \equiv \lim_{T \to \infty} \frac{|\hat{X}_T(\omega)|^2}{T} \quad . \tag{3.1.16}$$

In Figure 3.1.17 we display the power spectral densities (PSD) $S_{xx}(\omega)$ and $S_{zz}(\omega)$ as calculated by Farmer, Crutchfield, Froehling, Packard and Shaw (1980) using the trajectory shown. It is apparent from the power spectra density using the $X(t)$ time series that there is no dominant periodic $x-$component to the dynamics of the attractor, although lower frequencies are favored over higher ones. The power spectral density for the $Z(t)$ time series has a much flatter spectrum overall, but there are a few isolated frequencies at which energy is concentrated. This energy concentration would appear as a strong periodic component in the time trace of $Z(t)$. From these spectra one would conclude that $X(t)$ is non-periodic, but that $Z(t)$ possesses both periodic and non-periodic components. In fact from the linearity of the Fourier transform (3.1.15) we would say that $Z(t)$ is a superposition of these two parts:

$$Z(t) = Z_p(t) + Z_{np}(t) \quad . \tag{3.1.17}$$

The implication of (3.1.17) is that the auto-correlation function

$$C_{zz}(\tau) = \lim_{t \to \infty} \left\langle Z(t)Z(t+\tau) \right\rangle \tag{3.1.18}$$

may be written as the sum of a nonperiodic components $<Z_{np}(t)Z_{np}(t+\tau)>$ that decays to zero at $\tau \to \infty$ and a periodic component $<Z_p(t)Z_p(t+\tau)>$ that does not decay.

To summarize: we have here a new kind of attractor that is referred to as "strange" whose dynamics are "chaotic" and with a power spectra density resulting from the time series of the trajectory that has broadband components. Dynamical systems that are periodic or quasi-periodic have a PSD composed of delta functions, i.e., very narrow spectral peaks; non-periodic systems have broad spectra with no dramatic emphasis of any particular frequency. It is this broad band character of the PSD that is currently used to identify non-periodic behavior in experimental data.

So what does this all mean? In part what it means is that the dynamics of a complex system such as the brain or the heart might be random even if its description can be "isolated" to a few (three or more) degrees of freedom that interact in a deterministic but nonlinear way. If the system is dissipative, i.e., information is extracted from the system on the average, but the system is open to the environment, i.e., information is supplied to

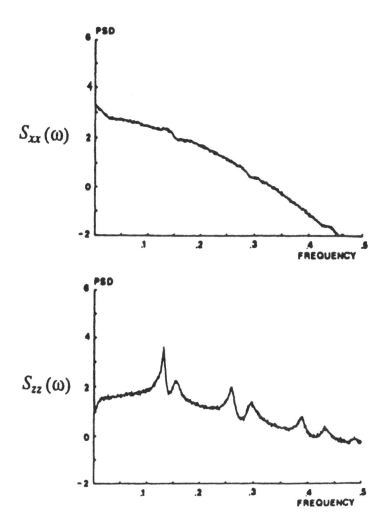

Figure 3.1.17.   The power spectral density $S_{xx}(\omega)$ and $S_{zz}(\omega)$ is calculated using the solution for the x-component and z-component, separately, using Equation (3.1.16) (from Farmer et al., 1980).

the system by means of boundary conditions, then a "strange attractor" is not only a possible manifold for the solutions to the dynamic equations; it, or something like it, may even be probable.

We show subsequently that the aperiodic or chaotic behavior of an attractor is a consequence of a sensitivity to initial conditions: trajectories that are initially nearby exponentially separate as they evolve forward in time on a chaotic attractor. Thus as Lorenz observed: microscopic perturbations (unobservable changes in the initial state of a system) are amplified to affect macroscopic behavior. This property is quite different from the qualitative features of nonchaotic attractors. In the latter, orbits that start out near one another remain close together forever. Thus small errors or perturbations remain bounded and the behavior of individual trajectories remain predictable.

As Crutchfield, Farmer, Packard and Shaw (1987) point out in their review *Chaos*, the key to understanding chaotic behavior lies in understanding a simple stretching and folding operation, which takes place in phase space [cf. Section (2.2)]. Recall that an attractor occupies a bounded region of phase space and that two initially nearby trajectories on a chaotic trajectory separate exponentially in time. But such a process of separation cannot continue indefinitely. In order to maintain both these properties the attractor must fold over onto itself like a taco. Thus although orbits diverge and follow increasingly different paths, they eventually come close together again but on different sections of the fold. As they explain, the orbits on a chaotic attractor are shuffled by this process of folding, much like a deck of cards is shuffled by a dealer. The unpredictability or randomness of the orbits on such an attractor is a consequence of this mixing process. The process of stretching and folding continues incessantly in the morphogenesis of the attractor, creating folds within folds ad infinitum. This means that such an attractor has structure on all scales, that is to say, *a chaotic attractor is a geometrically fractal object*. Thus, as we have discussed in the first chapter we would expect a strange attractor to have a noninteger dimension, i.e., a fractal dimension.

Of course these considerations are not of much practical value unless they can be implemented in the determination of the properties of a real data set. This will be done subsequently. The rationale for their application was also developed by Lorenz in his seminal work, but the full extent of its importance has only recently begun to emerge; see e.g. Lanford (1976). He (Lorenz) observed that the trajectory leaves the spiral centered at C say (see Figure 3.1.17), only after exceeding some critical distance from the center. Further, the degree to which this critical distance is exceeded determines the point at which the next spiral, i.e., that centered at C', is entered as well as the number of circuits executed prior to making the transition back to the C center again. Thus he concludes that "some single feature of a given circuit should predict the same feature of the following circuit." As an example he selected the maximum value of the $Z(t)$ variable along the trajectory which occurs whenever the circuit is nearly completed.

In Figure 3.1.18 the abscissa is labeled by the value of the nth maxima Z_n of $Z(t)$ and the ordinate is labeled by the value of the following maximum Z_{n+1}. It is clear that the points generated lie along a curve if the spaces between points are filled in. This is shown for example by Shaw (1981) using the increased computing capacity that has developed in the intervening years. The computer generated function clearly prescribe a two- to-one relation between Z_n and Z_{n+1}. From this relation one could formulate an empirical prediction scheme using the geometry of the attractor as a data set without a knowledge of the underlying dynamic equations. In the next section, after we learn about *mappings,* we will see how this is done.

A second example of a dynamic system whose solutions lie on a chaotic attractor was given by Rössler (1976) for a chemical process. He has in fact provided over half a dozen examples of such attractors [cf. Rössler (1978)], but we will not discuss all of them here. It is useful to consider his motivation for constructing such a variety of chaotic attractors. In large part it was to understand the detailed effects of the stretching and folding operations in nonlinear dynamical systems. These operations mix the orbits in phase space in the same way a baker mixes bread by kneading it, i.e., rolling it out and folding it over. Visualize a drop of red food coloring placed on top of a ball of dough. This red spot represents the initially nearby trajectories of a dynamic system. Now as the dough is rolled out for the first time the red spot is stretched into an ellipse, which eventually is folded over. After a sufficiently long time the red blob is stretch and folded many times, resulting in a ball of dough with alternating layers of red and white. Crutchfield et al. (1987) point out that after 20 such operations the initial blob has been stretched to more than a million times its original length, and its thickness has shrunk to the molecular level. The red dye is then thoroughly mixed with the dough, just as chaos thoroughly mixes the trajectories in phase space on the attractor.

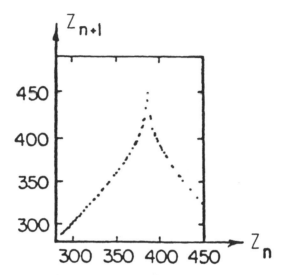

Figure 3.1.18.   Corresponding values of relative maximum of Z (abscissa) and subsequent relative maximum of Z (ordinate) occurring during the first 6000 iterations (from Lorenz, 1963).

The dynamic equations for Rössler's (1976) three degree of freedom system is

$$\dot{X} = -(Y + Z) \tag{3.1.19}$$

$$\dot{Y} = X + aY \tag{3.1.20}$$

$$\dot{Z} = b + XZ - cZ \;\; , \tag{3.1.21}$$

where a, b and c are constants. For one set of parameter values, Farmer et al. (1980) referred to the attractor as "the funnel," the obvious reason for this name is seen in Figure 3.1.19. Another set of parameter values yields the "simple Rössler attractor," (cf. Figure 3.1.20d). Both of these chaotic attractors have one positive Lyapunov exponent. As we mentioned earlier, a Lyapunov exponent is a measure of the rate at which trajectories separate one from the other (cf. Section 3.2). A negative exponent implies the orbits approach a common fixed point. A zero exponent means the orbits maintain their relative positions; they are on a stable attractor. Finally, a positive exponent implies the orbits exponentially separate; they are on a chaotic attractor. In Figure 3.1.20 we have depicted phase space projections of the attractor, just as we did for the Lorenz attractor.

Equations (3.1.19) - (3.1.21) is one of the simplest sets of differential equation models possessing a chaotic attractor. Figure 3.1.20 depicts a projection of the attractor onto the (x, y)-plane for four different values of the parameter c. Notice that as c is increased the trajectory changes from a simple limit cycle with a single maximum (Figure 3.1.20a), to one with two maxima (Figure 3.1.20b) and so on until finally the orbit becomes aperiodic (Figure 3.1.20d). Here again, as with the Lorenz attractor, we can relate the nth maximum of say $X(t)$ to the $(n+1)^{st}$ maximum. This can be done by noting the intersection of the trajectory in Figure 3.1.20 to a line placed transverse to the attractor. In this way we obtain the plot of the maximum shown in Figure 3.1.21, the curve yields the functional equation $x_{n+1} = f(x_n)$ which is a difference equation. This figure suggests how we can replace a continuous model by one which is discrete. We expand our discussion of this procedure in the following section.

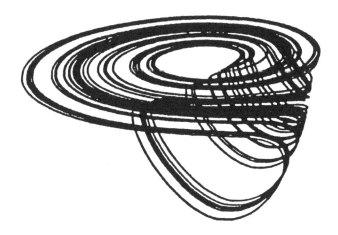

Figure 3.1.19. The "funnel" attractor solution to the Rössler Equations (3.1.19)-
(3.1.21) with parameter values $a = 0.343, b = 1.82$ and $c = 9.75$. (From
Rossler, 1979.)

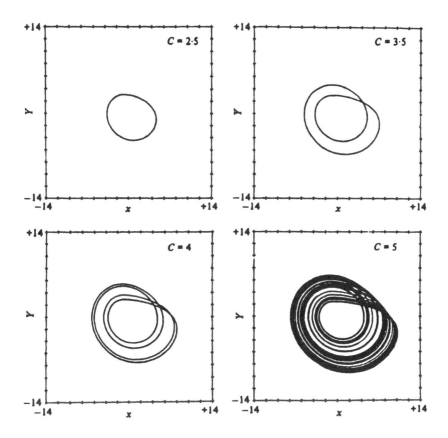

Figure 3.1.20.   An $x-y$ phase plane plot of the solution to the Rössler Equations
(3.1.19)-(3.1.21) with parameter values $a = 0.20$ and $b = 0.20$ at four
different values of c indicated in the graphs.

122

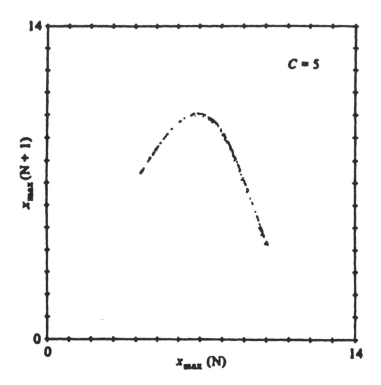

Figure 3.1.21.   Next amplitude plot of the Rössler Equations (3.1.19)-(3.1.21) for
$c = 5, a = 0.2$ and $b = 0.2$. Each amplitude of the oscillation of x was
plotted against the preceding amplitude.

3.2   Nonlinear Bio-Mapping

The modeling strategy adapted in the preceding section was essentially that which one finds throughout the physical sciences: construct continuous equations of evolution to describe the dynamics of the physical variable of interest. In physical systems one can use general principles such as the conservation of energy, or the conservation of action, or the conservation of momentum to construct such equations of motion. When this is not possible then one can employ reasonable physical arguments to construct the equations. In any event, once the equations of evolution have been specified, properties of the solutions are examined in great detail and compared with the known experimental properties of the physical system. It is the last stage, the comparison with data, that ultimately determines the veracity of the model dynamics. We have followed this procedure in broad outline in our discussion of the two coupled nonlinear oscillators modeling cardiac dynamics. In that discussion we were able to review a number of fundamental concepts in nonlinear dynamics that will prove useful subsequently.

Now that we have seen the brand of chaos associated with a continuous strange attractor, we examine a one-dimensional noninvertible nonlinear map. One of the fascinating aspect of these maps is that they appear to be the natural way in which to describe the time development of systems in which successive generations are quite distinct. Thus they are appropriate for describing the change in population levels between successive generations: in biology, where populations can refer to the number of individuals in a given species or the gene frequency of a mutation in an evolutionary model; in sociology , where population may refer to the number of people adopting the latest fad or fashion; in medicine, where the population is the number of individuals infected by a contagious disease; and so on. The result of the mathematical analysis is that for certain parameter regimes there are a large number of classes of discrete dynamical models (maps) with chaotic solutions. The *chaos* associated with these solutions is such that the orbits are periodic or erratic in time, and can be related to the chaos observed in the time series for strange attractors (cf. Chapter 4). Whether one describes the system's dynamics with a nonlinear map or whether the map arises from a projection of the dynamics from a higher dimensional space, they both indicate that one must abandon the notion that the deterministic nonlinear evolution of a process implies a predictable result. One may be able to solve the discrete equations of motion only to find a chaotic solution that requires a distribution function for making predictions.

124

In the present section we offer an alternative description of the evolution of biological systems from that adopted in Chapter 2; one which emphasizes the difference between physical and biological systems in a number of cases of interest. Just as in Section 3.1 we wish to describe the dynamics of a system characterized by an N-component vector $\mathbf{X} = (X_1, X_2, ..., X_N)$ and again in order to determine the future evolution of the system from its present state we must specify a dynamic rule for each of the components. For a great many biological and ecological systems the variables are not considered to be continuous functions of time, but rather as is the case of animal populations, to be functions of a discrete time index specifying successive generations. The minimum unit of time change for the dynamic equations would in this case be given by unity, i.e., the change of a single generation. Thus the equations of motion instead of being given by (3.1.1) would be of the form

$$\mathbf{X}(n+1) = \mathbf{F}\big[\mathbf{X}(n)\big] \qquad (3.2.1)$$

where the changes in the vector $\mathbf{X}(n)$ between generation n and $n+1$ is determined by the function $\mathbf{F}[\mathbf{X}(n)]$. If at generation $n = 0$ we specify the components of $\mathbf{X}(0)$, i.e., the set of circumstances characterizing the system, then the evolution of the system is determined by iteration (mapping) of the recursion relation (3.2.1) away from the initial state. Even in systems that are perhaps more properly described by continuous time equations of motion it is thought by many, see e.g. Collete and Eckmann (1980), that a discrete time representation may be used to isolate simplifying features of certain dynamical systems.

(a)   One-dimensional maps

The evolution equation in a discrete representation is called a *map* and the evolution is given by iterating the map, ie., by repeated application of the mapping operation to the newly generated points. Thus iterations of the form $X_n \rightarrow X_{n+1} = f(X_n)$, where f maps the one-dimensional interval [0, 1] onto itself, is interpreted as a discrete time version of a continuous dynamical system. The choice of interval [0, 1] is arbitrary since the change of variables $Y = (X-1)/(b-a)$ will replace a mapping of the interval $[a,b]$ into itself by one that maps [0, 1] into itself. For example, consider the continuous trajectory in the two-dimensional phase space depicted in Figure 3.2.1. The intersection points of

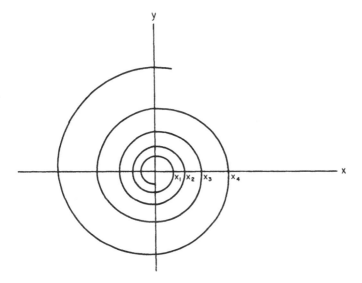

Figure 3.2.1. The spiral is an arbitrary orbit depicting a function $y = f(x)$. The intersection of the spiral with the x-axis defines a set of points $x_1, x_2, ...,$ that
can be obtained from a mapping determined by $f(x)$.

the orbit with the X-axis are denoted by $X_1, X_2, \cdots$. The point X_{n+1} can certainly be related to X_n by means of the function f determined by the trajectory. Thus, instead of solving the continuous differential equations that describe the trajectory, in this approach one produces models of the mapping function f and studies the properties of $X_{n+1} = f(X_n)$. Here, as we have said, n plays the role of the time variables. This strategy has been applied to models for biological, social, economic, chemical and physical systems. May (1976) has pointed out a number of possible applications of the fundamental equation for a single variable

$$X_{n+1} = f(X_n) \ . \tag{3.2.2}$$

In genetics, for example, X_n could describe the change in the gene frequency between successive generations; in epidemiology, the variable X_n could denote the fraction of the population infected at time n; in psychology, certain learning theories can be cast in the form where X_n is interpreted as the number of bits of information that can be remembered up to generation n; is sociology, X_n might be interpreted as the number of people having heard a rumor at time n and (3.2.2) would then describe the propagation of rumors in societies of various structures see, e.g., Kemeny and Snell (1972). The potential applications of such modeling equations are therefore restricted only by our imaginations.

Consider the simplest mapping, also called a recursion relation, in which a population X_n of organisms per unit area, on a petri dish for example, in the nth generation is strictly proportional to the population in the preceding generation with a proportionality constant μ:

$$X_n = \mu X_{n-1} \ , \quad n = 1, 2, \cdots . \tag{3.2.3}$$

The proportionality constant is given by the difference between the birth rate and death rate and is therefore the *net* birth rate of the population. Equation (3.2.3) is quite easy to solve. Suppose that the population has a level $X_0 = N_0$ at the initial generation, then the recursion relation yields the sequence of relation

$$X_1 = \mu N_0 \ , \quad X_2 = \mu X_1 = \mu^2 N_0 \ , \quad \cdots \tag{3.2.4}$$

so that in general

$$X_n = \mu^n N_0, \ n = 0,1,\cdots \ .$$

(3.2.5)

This rather simple solution already exhibits a number of interesting properties. Firstly, if the net birth rate μ is less than unity, then we can write $\mu^n = e^{-n\beta}$ where $\beta > 0$, so that the population decreases exponentially between successive generation (note $\beta = -\ln\mu$). This is a reflection of the fact that with $\mu < 1$, the population of organisms fails to reproduce itself from generation to generation and therefore it exponentially approaches extinction:

$$\lim_{n \to \infty} X_n = 0 \ \text{if} \ \mu < 1 \ .$$

(3.2.6)

On the other hand if $\mu > 1$, then we can write $\mu^n = e^{n\beta}$ where $\beta \ (=\ln\mu) > 0$, so the population increases exponentially from generation to generation. This is a reflection of the fact that with $\mu > 1$ the population has an excess at each generation resulting in a population explosion. This is the Malthus' exponential population growth:

$$\lim_{n \to \infty} X_n = \infty \ \text{if} \ \mu > 1 \ .$$

(3.2.7)

The only value of μ for which the population does not have these extreme tendencies is $\mu = 1$, when, since the population reproduces itself exactly in each generation, we obtain the unstable situation:

$$\lim_{n \to \infty} X_n = N_0 \ .$$

(3.2.8)

Of course this simple model is no more valid than the continuous growth law of Malthus (1798), which he used to describe the exponential growth of human populations. It is curious that the modeling of such growth, although attributed to Malthus did not originate with him. In fact Malthus was an economist and clergyman interested in the moral implications of such population growth. His contribution to population dynamics was the exploration of the consequences of the fact that a geometrically growing population will always outstrip a linearly growing food supply, resulting in overcrowding and misery. Why the food supply should grow linearly was never questioned by him. A more scientifically oriented investigator, Verhulst (1844), put forth a theory that somewhat mediated the pessimistic view of Malthus. Verhulst noted that the growth of real populations is not unbounded. He argued that such factors as the availability of food, shelter, sanitary conditions, etc. all restrict (or at least influence) the growth of populations. He included these effects by making the growth rate μ a function of the population level. His arguments allows us to generalize the discrete model to include the effects of limited resources. In particular, the birthrate is assumed to decrease with increasing population in a linear way:

$$\mu \to \mu(X_n) = \mu[1 - X_n/\Theta] \quad , \tag{3.2.9}$$

where Θ is the saturation level of the population. Thus the linear recursion relation (3.2.3) is replaced with the nonlinear discrete *logistic equation* ,

$$X_{n+1} = \mu X_n [1 - X_n/\Theta] \quad . \tag{3.2.10}$$

It is clear that when $X_n << \Theta$ the population grows exponentially since the nonlinear term is negligible. However at some point the ratio X_n/Θ is going to be of the order unity and the rate of population growth will be retarded. When $X_n = \Theta$ there are no more births in the population. Biologically the regime $X_n > \Theta$ corresponds to a negative birthrate, but this does not make biological sense and so we restrict the region of *interpretation* of this model to $[1 - X_n/\Theta] > 0$. Finally, we reduce the number of parameters from two, μ and Θ, to one by introducing $Y_n = X_n/\Theta$ the fraction of the saturation level achieved by the population. In terms of this *ratio* variable the recursion relation (3.2.10) becomes

$$Y_{n+1} = \mu Y_n [1 - Y_n] \quad . \tag{3.2.11}$$

Segal (1984) challenges the readers of his book (at this point in the analysis of this mapping) to attempt and predict the type of behavior manifest by the solution to (3.2.11), e.g. Are there periodic components to the solution? Does extinction ever occur?, etc. His intent was to alert the reader to the inherent complexity contained in the deceptively simple looking equation (3.2.11). We will examine some of these general properties shortly, but first let us explore our example a bit more fully. Our intent is to introduce the reader to a number of fundamental dynamical concepts that will be useful in the subsequent study of biomedical data.

We noticed that extinction was the solution to the simple system (3.2.3) when $\mu < 1$. Is extinction a possible solution to (3.2.11)? If it is, then once that state is attained, it must remain unchanged throughout the remaining generations. Put differently, extinction must be a *steady-state solution* of the recursion relation. A steady-state solution is one for which $Y_n = Y_{n+1}$ for all n. Let us assume the existence of a steady-state level Y_{ss} of the population such that (3.2.11) becomes

$$Y_{ss} = \mu Y_{ss}(1 - Y_{ss}) \qquad (3.2.12)$$

for all n, since in the steady-state $Y_{n+1} = Y_n = Y_{ss}$. Equation (3.2.12) defines the quadratic equation

$$Y_{ss}^2 + (1/\mu - 1) Y_{ss} = 0 , \qquad (3.2.13)$$

which has the two roots $Y_{ss} = 0$, and $Y_{ss} = (1 - 1/\mu)$. The $Y_{ss} = 0$ root corresponds to extinction, but we now have a second steady solution to the mapping, that being $Y_{ss} = 1-1/\mu$ which is positive for $\mu > 1$. One of the questions that is of interest in the more general treatment of this problem is to determine to which of these steady states the population evolves as the years go by, i.e., extinction or some finite constant level.

Before we examine the more general properties of (3.2.11) and equations like it, let us use a more traditional tool of analysis and examine the stability of the two steady states found above. Traditionally the stability of a system in the vicinity of a given value is determined by perturbation theory. We use that technique now and write

$$Y_n = Y_{ss} + \xi_n , \qquad (3.2.14)$$

where $\xi_n << Y_{ss}$ so that (3.2.14) denotes a small change in the relative population from its steady-state value. If we now substitute (3.2.14) into (3.2.11) we obtain

$$Y_{ss} + \xi_{n+1} = \mu(Y_{ss} + \xi_n)\left[1 - Y_{ss} - \xi_n\right] . \qquad (3.2.15)$$

Then using (3.2.12) to eliminate certain terms and neglecting terms quadratic in ξ_n we obtain

$$\xi_{n+1} = (\mu - 2Y_{ss}) \xi_n \qquad (3.2.16)$$

as the recursion relation for the perturbation. In the neighborhood of extinction, the $Y_{ss} = 0$ steady state, (3.2.16) reduces to (3.2.3) in the variable ξ_n rather than X_n. Therefore if $0 < \mu < 1$ then the fixed point $Y_{ss} = 0$ is stable and if $\mu > 1$ the fixed point is unstable. By stable we mean that $\xi_n \to 0$ as $n \to \infty$ if $0 < \mu < 1$ so that the system returns to the fixed point, i.e., ξ_n decreases exponentially in n. By unstable we mean that $\xi_n \to \infty$ as

$n \to \infty$ if $\mu > 1$ so that the perturbation grows without bound and never returns to the fixed point, i.e., ξ_n increases exponentially with n. Of course $\mu = 1$ means the fixed point is neutrally stable, i.e., it neither return to nor diverges from $Y_{ss} = 0$. It is also clear that in the unstable case that the condition for perturbation theory will eventually break down as ξ_n increases. When this occurs more sophisticated analysis is required.

In the neighborhood of the steady state $Y_{ss} = 1 - 1/\mu$ the recursion relation becomes

$$\xi_{n+1} = (2 - \mu)\xi_n \quad . \tag{3.2.17}$$

The preceding analysis can again be repeated with the result that if $1 > 2 - \mu > -1$ the fixed point $Y_{ss} = 1 - 1/\mu$ is stable and implies that the birthrate is in the interval $1 < \mu < 3$. The stability is monotonic for $1 < \mu < 2$, but because of the changes in sign it is oscillatory for $2 < \mu < 3$. Similarly the fixed point is unstable for $0 < \mu < 1$ (monotonic) and $\mu > 3$ (oscillatory).

Following Olsen and Degn (1985) we examine the nature of the solutions to (3.2.11) as a function of the parameter μ a bit more closely. This can be done using a simple computer code to evaluate the iterates Y_n. For $0 < \mu \le 4$ insert an initial value $0 \le Y_0 \le 1$ into (3.2.11) and generate a Y_1, which is also in the interval [0, 1]. This second value of the iterate is then inserted back into (3.2.11) and a third value Y_2 is generated; here again $0 \le Y_2 \le 1$. This process of generation and reinsertion constitutes the dynamic process, which is a mapping of the unit interval into itself in a two- to-one manner, i.e., two values of the iterate at step n can be used to generate a particular value of the iterate at step $n+1$. In Figure 3.2.2a we show Y_n as a function of n for $\mu = 2.8$ and observe that as n becomes large ($n > 10$) the value of Y_n becomes constant. This value is a fixed point of the mapping equal to $1 - 1/\mu = 0.643$, and is approached by all initial conditions $0 < Y_0 < 1$ i.e., it is an attractor. Quite a different behavior is observed for the same initial point when $\mu = 3.2$. In Figure 3.2.2b we see that after an initial transient the process becomes periodic, that is to say that the iterate alternates between two values. This periodic orbit is called a 2-cycle. Thus, the fixed point becomes unstable at the parameter value $\mu = 3$ and bifurcates into a 2-cycle. Here the 2-cycle becomes the attractor for

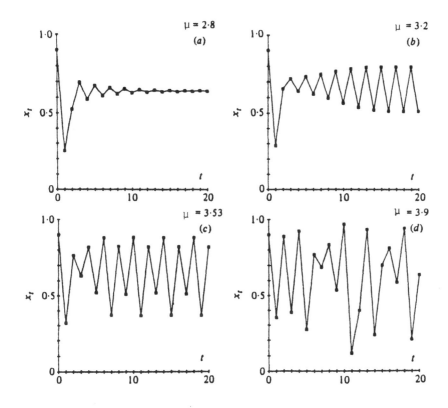

Figure 3.2.2. The solution to the map (3.2.11) is depicted for various choices of the parameter μ. (a) The solution Y_n approaches a constant value as $n \rightarrow \infty$ for $\mu = 2.8$. (b) The solution Y_n is a periodic orbit after the initial transient dies out for $\mu = 3.2$. (c) The orbit in (b) bifurcates to a 4-cycle for $\mu = 3.53$. (d) The orbit is chaotic for $\mu = 3.9$. (From Olsen and Degn, 1985.)

the mapping. For a slightly larger value of μ, $\mu = 3.53$, the mapping settles down into a pattern in which the value of the iterate alternates between two large values and two small values (cf. Figure 3.2.2c). Here again the existing orbit, a 2-cycle, has become unstable at $\mu = 3.444$ and bifurcated into a 4-cycle. Thus, we see that as μ is increased a fixed point changes into a 2-cycle, a 2-cycle changes into a 4-cycle, which in turn will change into an 8-cycle and so on. This process of period doubling is called subharmonic bifurcation since a cycle of a given frequency ω_0 bifurcates into periodic orbits which are subharmonics of the original orbit, i.e., for k bifurcations the frequency of the orbit is $\omega_0/2^k$. The attractor for the dynamic process can therefore be characterized by the appropriate values of μ.

As one might have anticipated, the end point of this period doubling process is an orbit with an infinite period (zero frequency). An infinite period implies that the system is áperiodic, that is to say, the pattern of the values of the iterate does not repeat itself in any finite number of iterations, i.e., finite time interval (cf. Figure 3.2.2d). We have already seen that any process that does not repeat itself as time goes to infinity is completely unique and hence is random. It was this similarity of the mapping to discrete random sequences that motivated the coining of the term chaotic to describe such attractors. The deterministic mapping (3.2.11) can therefore generate chaos for certain values of the parameter μ.

Returning now to the more general context it may appear that limiting the present analysis to one-dimensional systems is unduly restrictive; however, we recall that the system is pictured to be a projection of a more complicated dynamical system onto a one-dimensional subspace (cf. e.g. Figure 3.2.1). A substantial literature based on (3.2.11) has developed in the past decade, much of which is focused on the purely mathematical properties of such mappings. We are not concerned with that vast literature here, except insofar as it makes available to us solutions and insights that can be applied in *biology* and *medicine*. The physicists and mathematicians have been quite actively exploring the consequences of these results for physical and chemical systems, but with a few notable exceptions activity in the other sciences has been relatively subdued (cf. Chapter 4).

One of the exceptions alluded to is the remarkable review article of May in which he makes clear the state of the art in discrete systems up until 1976. In addition he makes the following comments:

> "The review ends with an evangelical plea for the introduction of these difference equations into elementary mathematics courses, so that students intuitions may be enriched by seeing the wild things that simple nonlinear equations can do."

His plea was motivated by the recognition that the traditional mathematical tools such as Fourier analysis, orthogonal functions, etc. are all fundamentally linear and

> "...the mathematical intuition so developed ill equips the students to confront the bizarre behavior exhibited by the simplest discrete nonlinear systems, ... Yet such nonlinear systems are surely the rule, not the exceptions, outside the physical sciences."

May ends his article with the following indictment:

> "Not only in research, but also in the everyday world of politics and economics, we would all be better off if more people realized that simple systems do not necessarily possess simple dynamic properties."

For the moment we shall make the assumption that the maps (discrete dynamical systems) of interest contain a single maximum and that $f(X)$ is monotonically increasing for values of X below this maximum and monotonically decreasing for values of X above this maximum. Maps such as these, i.e., maps with a single maximum, are called noninvertible, since, given X_{n+1} there are two possible values of X_n and therefore the functional relation cannot be inverted. If the index n is interpreted as the discrete time variable, as we did above, the recursion relation generates new values of X_n forward in time but not backward in time, see e.g. Ott (1985). This assumption corresponds to the reasonable requirement that the dynamic law stimulates X to grow when it is near zero, but inhibits its growth when it reaches some saturation value. An example of this is provided by the discrete version of the Verhulst equation for population growth that we have just examined. Equation (3.2.10) is often called the discrete logistic equation and has been intensively studied in the physical sciences, usually in the scaled form (3.2.11). Thus the mapping function is $f(Y_n) = \mu Y_n (1 - Y_n)$ and when graphed versus Y_n yields the quadratic curve depicted in Figure 3.2.3.

134

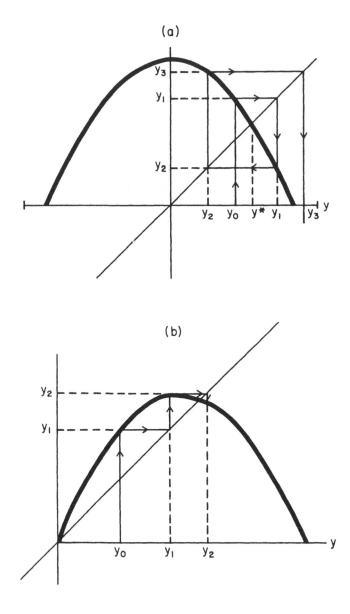

Figure 3.2.3. A mapping function with a single maximum is shown. In (a), the iteration
away from the initial point y_0 is depicted. In (b), the convergence to the
station point y^* is shown. (From West, 1985.)

The mapping operation is one that is accomplished by applying the function f to a given initial values Y_0 to generate the next point, and applied sequentially to generate the successive images of this point. The point Y_n is generated by applying the mapping f, n times to the initial point Y_0:

$$Y_n = f^n(Y_0) \qquad (3.2.18)$$

using the relation $f^n(Y_0) = f[f^{n-1}(Y_0)]$. This is done graphically in Figure 3.2.3a for $n = 3$ using the rule: starting from the initial point Y_0 a line is drawn to the function yielding the value $Y_1 = f(Y_0)$ along the ordinate, then from symmetry the same value is obtained along the abscissa by drawing a line to the diagonal (45°) line. An application of f to Y_1 is then equivalent to dropping a line from the diagonal to the f-curve to yield $Y_2 = f(Y_1) = f[f(Y_0)] = f^2(Y_0)$. The value Y_3 is obtained in exactly the same way from $Y_3 = f^3(Y_0)$. The intersection of the diagonal with the function f defines a point Y^* having the property

$$Y^* = f(Y^*) \qquad (3.2.19)$$

which is called a *fixed point* of the dynamic equation, i.e., Y^* is the Y_{ss} from (3.2.12). The fixed points correspond to the steady-state solutions of the discrete equation and for (3.2.11) there are $Y^* = 1 - 1/\mu$ (nontrivial) and $Y^* = 0$ (trivial). We can see in Figure 3.2.3b that the iterated points are approaching Y^* and as $n \rightarrow \infty$ they will reach this fixed point. To determine if a mapping will approach a fixed point asymptotically, i.e., if the fixed point is stable, we examine the slope of the function at the fixed point, see e.g., May (1976); Li and Yorke (1975); Collet and Eckmann (1980). The function acts like a curved mirror either focusing the ray towards the fixed point under multiple reflections or diverging the ray away. The asymptotic direction (either towards or away from the fixed point) is determined by the slope of the function at Y^*, which is depicted in Figure 3.2.4 by the dashed line and denoted by $f'(Y^*)$, i.e., the (tangent) derivative of $f(Y)$ at $Y = Y^*$. As long as $|f'(Y^*)| < 1$ the iterations of the map are attracted to $Y = Y^*$, just as the perturbation ξ approaches zero in (3.2.14) near the stable fixed point. Again using a logistic map as an example, we have $f'(Y^*) = 2 - \mu$, so that the equilibrium point is stable and attracts all trajectories originating in the interval $0 < Y < 1$ if and only if $1 < \mu < 3$. This is of course the same result we obtained using linear stability theory [cf. Eq. (3.2.17)] for the logistic map.

136

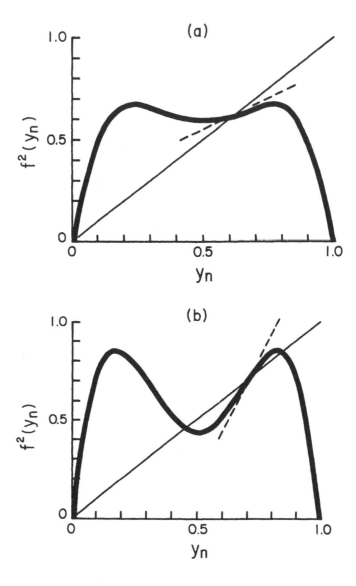

Figure 3.2.4. The map f with a single maximum in Figure 3.2.3 yields an f^2 map with a double maximum. The slope at the point y^* is indicated by the dashed line and is seen to increase as the parameter μ is raised in the map from (a) to (b). (From West, 1985.)

When the slope of f is such that the fixed point becomes unstable, i.e., when $|f'(Y^*)|>1$, then the solution "spirals" out. If the parameter μ is continuously increased until this instability is reached then the orbit will spiral out until it encounters a situation where $Y_2^* = f(Y_1^*)$ and $Y_1^* = f(Y_2^*)$, i.e., the orbit becomes periodic. Said differently, the mapping f has a *periodic orbit* of period 2 since $Y_2^* = f(Y_1^*) = f^2(Y_2^*)$ and $Y_1^* = f(Y_2^*) = f^2(Y_1^*)$ since Y_1^* and Y_2^* are fixed points of the mapping f^2 and not of the mapping f. In Figure 3.2.4a we illustrate the mapping f^2 and observe it to have two maxima rather than the single one of f. As the parameter μ is increased further the dimple between the two maxima increases as do the height of the peaks along with the slopes of the intersection of f^2 with the diagonal (cf. Figure 3.2.4b).

For $1<\mu<3$ the fixed point is stable and Y^* is a degenerate fixed point of f^2, i.e., $Y^* = f^2(Y^*)$. At $\mu = 3.414$ the fixed point becomes unstable and two new solutions to the quadratic mapping emerge. These are the two intersections of the quadratic map with the diagonal having slopes with magnitude less than unity, Y_1^* and Y_2^*. The chain rule of differentiation of the derivative of f^2 at Y_1^* and Y_2^* is the product of the derivatives along the periodic orbit

$$f^{2\prime}(Y_1^*) = f'[f(Y_1^*)]f'(Y_1^*) = f'(Y_1^*)f'(Y_2^*) = f^{2\prime}(Y_2^*) \qquad (3.2.20)$$

so that the slope is the same at both points of the period 2 orbit, see e.g. Li and Yorke (1975), and in fact the slope is the same at all k of the values of a period k orbit. This is in fact a continuous process starting from the stable fixed point Y^* when $|f'|<1$; as μ is increased this point becomes unstable at $|f'| = 1$ and generates two new stable points with $|f^{2\prime}|<1$ for a period 2 orbit; as μ is increased further these points become unstable at $|f^{2\prime}| = 1$ and generates four new stable points with $|f^{4\prime}|<1$ for a period 4 orbit. This bifurcation sequence is tied to the value of the parameter μ. As this parameter is increased the discrete equation undergoes a sequence of bifurcations from the fixed point to stable cycles with periods 2, 4, 8, 16, 32 ... 2^k. In each case the bifurcation process is the same as that for the transition from the stable fixed point to the stable period 2 orbit. A graph indicating the location of the stable values of Y for a given μ is given in Figure 3.2.5. Here we see that the μ interval between successive bifurcations is diminishing so that the "window" of values of μ wherein any one cycle is stable progressively diminishes. If we denote by μ_k the value of μ where the orbit bifurcates from length 2^{k-1} to

138

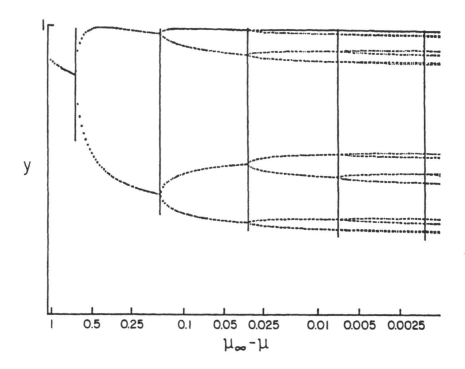

Figure 3.2.5. The bifurcation of the solution to the mapping $x \to 1 - \mu x^2$ as a function of $\mu_\infty - \mu$ is indicated. The logarithmic scale was chosen to clearly depict the bifurcation regions. (From Collett and Eckmann, 1980.)

2^k, then

$$\lim_{k \to \infty} \frac{\mu_k - \mu_{k-1}}{\mu_{k+1} - \mu_k} = \text{universal constant} , \qquad (3.2.21)$$

a result first obtained numerically by Feigenbaum (1979). This result indicates that a constant μ_∞ is being approached by this sequence. This critical parameter value is a point of accumulation of a period 2^k cycles. For (3.2.11) the critical value of this parameter is $\mu_\infty = 3.5700$. The numerical value of μ_∞ is dependent on the particular map considered, although the existence of an accumulation point does not, and more importantly the universal constant in (3.2.21) has a value 4.69210 ... and is also independent of the specific choice of the map.

In Figure 3.2.5 we use the logarithm of μ as the abscissa in order to clearly distinguish the bifurcation points. In Figure 3.2.6 we replot this sequence linearly in μ. In the latter figure we distinguish from left to right, a stable fixed point, orbit of period 1; a stable orbit of period 2, then 4, 8 and then a haze of orbits starting along the line μ_∞, then another orbit of period 6 then 5, and 3. Collet and Eckmann (1980) comment: "The astonishing fact about this arrangement of stable periodic orbits is its *independence* of the particular one-parameter family of maps." The haze of points beyond μ_∞ consists of an infinite number of fixed points with different periodicities, along with an infinite number of different periodic orbits. In addition there are an uncountable number of aperiodic trajectories (bounded) each of which is associated with a different initial point Y_0. Two such adjacent initial points generate orbits that become arbitrarily distant with iteration number; no matter how long the time series generated by $f(Y)$ is iterated, the two patterns never repeat. As mentioned, Li and Yorke (1975) have applied the term *chaotic* to this hazy region where an infinite number of different trajectories can occur.

Thus we have arrived at the remarkable fact that a simple discrete deterministic equation can generate trajectories that are aperiodic. In particular in order to form a one-dimensional map to exhibit chaotic behavior, it must be noninvertible. May (1976) points out a number of practical implications of this result. The first being

"... that the apparently random fluctuation in census data for an animal population need not necessarily betoken either the vagaries of an unpredictable environment or sampling errors: they may simply derive from a rigidly deterministic population growth relationship such as (3.2.11)."

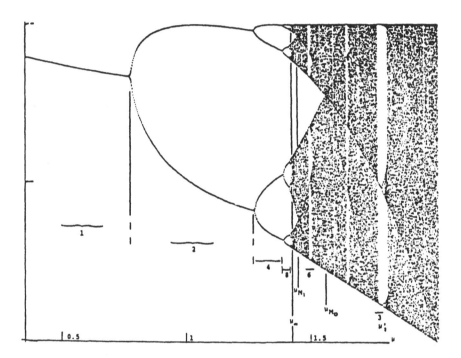

Figure 3.2.6.   The same as Figure 3.2.5, but with a linear scale in $\mu_\infty - \mu$ so that the hazy region denoting chaos is clearly observed. (From Collett and Eckmann, 1980.)

(b)   **Two-dimensional maps**

In the above discussion we defined a mapping in terms of a projection of a higher order dynamic system onto a one-dimensional line. This same definition can be applied for the intersection of the trajectories of a higher order dynamic process with a two-dimensional plane. In Figure 3.2.7 a sketch of a trajectory in three dimensions is shown, the intersection of the orbit with a plane defines a set of points that can be obtained by means of the two-dimensional map:

$$X_{n+1} = f_1(X_n, Y_n) \ , \ \ Y_{n+1} = f_2(X_n, Y_n) \ . \tag{3.2.22}$$

Here we follow Ott (1985) and consider only invertible maps where (3.2.22) can be solved uniquely for X_n and Y_n as functions of X_{n+1} and Y_{n+1}; $X_n = g_1(X_{n+1}, Y_{n+1})$ and $Y_n = g_2(X_{n+1}, Y_{n+1})$. If n is the time index then invertibility is equivalent to time reversibility, so that these maps are reversible in time whereas those in the preceding discussion were not. The maps in this section are analogous to the Hamiltonian dynamic equations discussed in physics and chemistry and not the dissipative equations leading to the strange attractors such as the Lorenz model.

The reason for examining higher order maps, such as the two-dimensional example given by (3.2.22) is that under certain conditions these maps have many of the properties of the so called strange attractors discussed earlier even though they are conservative. Thus we may anticipate that complex systems in the biological and behavioral sciences for which discrete equations may be a more natural way to model the dynamics than would be the traditional continuous equations of the physical science, do not have to be reduced to one-dimensional maps in order to see chaos emerge. In particular we establish the connection between these invertible maps and the strange attractor of Lorenz as well as to the fractal dimension discussed earlier.

The one-dimensional noninvertible maps were obtained by projecting a higher order trajectory onto a one-dimensional line. Let us now reverse the process and expand the space of the noninvertible map from one to two dimensions by introducing the coordinate Y_n in the following way:

$$X_{n+1} = f(X_n) + Y_n \tag{3.2.23}$$

$$Y_{n+1} = \beta X_n \ . \tag{3.2.24}$$

Of course, if f is noninvertible and $\beta = 0$ (3.2.23) collapses back onto the one-

142

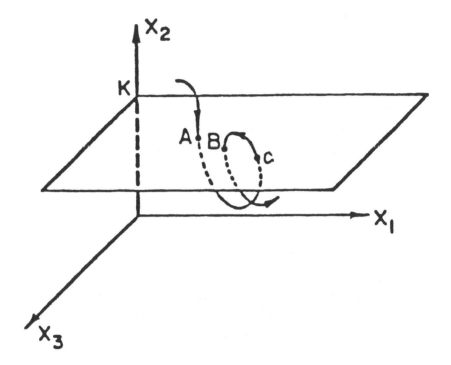

Figure 3.2.7. An arbitrary trajectory is shown and its intersection with a plane parallel to the x_1, x_3 – plane at $x_2 = constant$ are recorded. The points A, B, C,... define a map as in Figure 3.2.1. This is the Poincaré surface of section. (From Ott, 1985.)

dimensional map (3.2.11). For any non-zero β, however, the map (3.2.23) is invertible, i.e., $X_n = Y_{n+1}/\beta$ and $Y_n = X_{n+1} - f(Y_{n+1}/\beta)$. Thus we have transformed a noninvertible map to an invertible one by extending the space. As Ott (1985) points out, however, if β is sufficiently small the distinction between the invertible two-dimensional map and the noninvertible one-dimensional map may not be measurable.

Let us examine the behavior of a small phase space volume as the two-dimensional map is iterated from $X_n Y_n = V_n$ to $X_{n+1} Y_{n+1} = V_{n+1}$ in analogy to what was done with the Lorenz model. Recall that for the Lorenz attractor a small phase space volume obtained by perturbing the solutions of the equations of motion contracted due to dissipation. Here the relation between the two volumes V_n and V_{n+1} is

$$V_{n+1} = JV_n \qquad (3.2.25)$$

where J is the Jacobian of the map:

$$J \equiv \begin{vmatrix} \dfrac{\partial X_{n+1}}{\partial X_n} & \dfrac{\partial X_{n+1}}{\partial Y_n} \\[2ex] \dfrac{\partial Y_{n+1}}{\partial X_n} & \dfrac{\partial Y_{n+1}}{\partial Y_n} \end{vmatrix} \qquad (3.2.26)$$

Inserting (3.2.23) and (3.2.24) into (3.2.26) we find $J = -\beta$ so that the volume at consecutive times (3.2.25) is given by

$$V_{n+1} = -\beta V_n \qquad (3.2.27)$$

which for an initial volume V_0 has the solution

$$V_{n+1} = (-1)^{n+1} \beta^{n+1} V_0 \ , \qquad (3.2.28)$$

so that if $|\beta| < 1$ the volume will contract by a factor $|\beta|$ at each application of the mapping. As in the continuous case this contraction does *not* imply that the solution goes over to a point in phase space, but only that it is attracted to some bounded region of dimension lower than that of the initial phase space. If the dimension of the attractor is non-integer, then the attractor is fractal; see e.g. in Mandelbrot (1980) where the observation that the fractal dimension of a set may or may not be consistent with the term *strange*. Following Eckmann (1981), we employ the property that, if all the points in the initial volume V_0 converge to a single attractor, but that points which are arbitrarily close initially separate exponentially in time, then that attractor is called strange. This property of nearby trajectories to exponentially separate in time is called *sensitive dependence on initial conditions* and gives rise to the áperiodic behavior of strange attractors. There exists however a large variety of attractors which are neither periodic orbits nor fixed points and which are not strange attractors. All of these, states Eckmann (1981), seem to present more or less pronounced chaotic features. Thus there are attractors that are erratic but not strange. We will not pursue this general class here.

As an example of the two-dimensional invertible mapping we first transform the logistic equation (3.2.1) into the family of maps $X_{n+1} = 1 - cX_n^2$ with the parametric identification $c = (\mu/2 - 1)\mu/2$ and $0 < c \leq 2$, since $2 < \mu \leq 4$ and X_n maps the interval $[-1, 1]$ onto itself. Then using (3.2.23) and (3.2.24) we obtain the mapping first studied by Henon[61]

$$X_{n+1} = 1 - cX_n^2 + Y_n \qquad (3.2.29)$$

$$Y_{n+1} = \beta X_n \cdot \qquad (3.2.30)$$

In Figure 3.2.8 we have copied the loci of points for the Henon system in which 10^4 successive points from the mapping with the parameter values $c = 1.4$ and $\beta = 0.2$ initiated from a variety of choice of (X_0, Y_0). Ott (1985) points out that, as the map is iterated, points come closer and closer to the attractor eventually becoming indistinguishable from it. This, however, is an illusion of scale. If the mixed-in region of the figure is magnified one obtains Figure 3.2.9a from which a great deal of structure of the attractor can be discerned. If the boxed region in this latter figure is magnified, then what had appeared as three unequally spaced lines appear in Figure 3.2.9b as three distinct parallel intervals containing structure. Notice that the region in the box of Figure 3.2.9a appears the same as that in Figure 3.2.9b. Magnifying the boxed region in this latter region we obtain Figure 3.2.9c, which aside from resolution is a self-similar representation of the structure seen on the two preceding scales. Thus we observe scale invariant, Cantor-set-like structure transverse to the linear structure of the attractor. Ott (1985) concludes that because of this self-similar structure the attractor is probably strange. In fact it has been verified by direct calculation that initially nearby points separate exponentially in time (see e.g. Feit, 1978; Curry, 1979), thereby coinciding with at least one definition of a strange attractor.

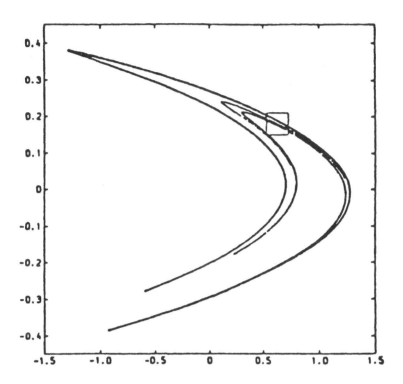

Figure 3.2.8. Iterated point of the map (3.2.2a), for 10^4 iterations with the parameter values $c = 1.4$ and $\beta = 0.2$. (From Ott, 1985.)

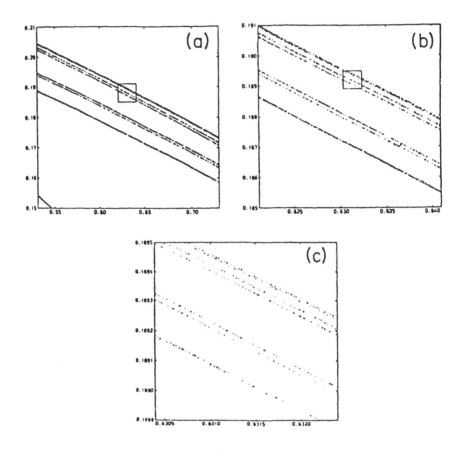

Figure 3.2.9. (a) Enlargement of the boxed region in Figure 3.2.8, 10^4 iterations; (b) enlargement of the square in (a), 10^6 iterations; (c) enlargement of the square in (b), 5×10^6 iterations. (From Ott, 1985.)

(c)   The Lyapunov exponent

We have adopted the definition that chaotic systems are those that have a sensitive dependence on initial conditions. This sensitivity requires that orbits initially near to one another exponentially separate as they evolve forward in time. A computable quantitative measure of the rate at which orbits separate is the Lyapunov exponent. For a one-dimensional map the Lyapunov exponent is defined by the slope of the map:

$$\sigma = \lim_{n \to \infty} \frac{1}{N} \sum_{n=1}^{N} ln \; |\frac{df \, (Y_n)}{dY}| \qquad (3.2.31)$$

where $Y_{n+1} = f \, (Y_n)$. Shaw (1981) has shown that σ is also the *average* information change over the entire interval of iteration. He argues that a map may be interpreted as a machine that takes a single input Y_0 and generates a string of numbers during the iteration process. If the string has a pattern such as would arise for an attractor that is a fixed point or periodic orbit, then after a very short time the machines gives *no new information*. On the other hand if the orbit is chaotic so that the string of numbers is random, then each iterate is new to the observer, and gives a new piece of information. Shaw convincingly demonstrates that a chaotic process is a generator of information. He argues that a negative σ implies a periodic orbit and the magnitude of σ measures the degree of stability of that orbit against perturbations. If an orbit is initiated at a point off the periodic orbit, but within its basin of attraction, the initial data will be lost as the orbit damps to its stable values. The parameter σ determines the rate at which this information is lost to the macroscopic world. If σ is positive, then it determines the rate of divergence of nearby trajectories which is the same as the rate of information production; see Oseledec (1968).

As an example let us take $\mu = 4$ in (3.2.11). Then if we define a new variable

$$Z_n = \frac{2}{\pi} \; sin^{-1} \, (\sqrt{Y_n} \,) \qquad (3.2.32)$$

the logistic map transforms to the "tent map"

$$Z_{n+1} = \begin{cases} 2Z_n & 0 \le Y_n \le 0.5 \\ 2(1 - Z_n) & 0.5 \le Y_n \le 1 \end{cases} \cdot \qquad (3.2.33)$$

From this we obtain for the slope of the map to be used in (3.2.31)

$$\left| \frac{df \, (Z_n)}{dZ} \right| = 2 \qquad (3.2.34)$$

for all Z, so that

$$\sigma = \ln 2 \approx 0.693 > 0 \ . \tag{3.2.35}$$

Since this quantity is *invariant* under coordinate transformations this proves that the logistic map with $\mu = 4$ meets our definition of a chaotic dynamical system, i.e., 0.693 bits of information are generated in each iteration. In fact this mapping is chaotic for all $\sigma > \sigma_\infty = 3.57 \cdots$ since $\sigma > 0$ for all these values.

Let us consider an N-dimensional map, i.e., $\mathbf{X} = (X^1, X^2, \ldots, X^N)$,

$$\mathbf{X}_{n+1} = \mathbf{f}(\mathbf{X}_n) \tag{3.2.36}$$

for which we have a trajectory $\mathbf{X}'_n$ in this phase space with initial condition $\mathbf{X}_0$ and a nearby trajectory $\mathbf{X}_n$ with initial condition $\mathbf{X}_0 + \Delta\mathbf{X}_0$ and $\|\Delta\mathbf{X}_0\| << \|\mathbf{X}_0\|$. Here the double bars denote the norm of the vector. The difference between the two trajectories $\Delta\mathbf{X}_0$ defines the tangent vector $\mathbf{u}_n \equiv \Delta\mathbf{X}_n$ such that (3.2.36) can be used to write

$$\mathbf{u}_{n+1} = \mathbf{f}(\mathbf{X}'_n) - \mathbf{f}(\mathbf{X}_n) \quad \cong \quad \frac{\partial\mathbf{f}}{\partial\mathbf{X}} \cdot \mathbf{u}_n + \cdots \tag{3.2.37}$$

which defines the linearized mapping

$$\mathbf{u}_{n+1} = \mathbf{A}(\mathbf{X}_n) \cdot \mathbf{u}_n \ . \tag{3.2.38}$$

where $\mathbf{A}$ is the $N \times N$ matrix defined by

$$\mathbf{A}(\mathbf{X}_n) = \frac{\partial}{\partial\mathbf{X}} \mathbf{f}(\mathbf{X}_n) \tag{3.2.39}$$

so that the map (3.2.38) is linearized along the trajectory $\mathbf{X}_n$. Following Nicolis (1986) the solution to (3.2.38) for a given initial condition $\hat{\mathbf{e}}_0$ at the nth iteration can be written as

$$\mathbf{u}_n = U_{n,n-1} U_{n-1,n-2} \cdots U_{21} U_{10} \hat{\mathbf{e}}_0 \ , \tag{3.2.40}$$

where $\mathbf{U}$ is the fundamental solution matrix. The indexing on $\mathbf{U}$ indicates the iteration for which it is the solution to the mapping. Let us interpret (3.2.40) starting with the right-most factor: $U_{10}\hat{\mathbf{e}}_0 = \mathbf{u}_1$, is the solution (3.2.38) for the initial condition $\mathbf{X}_0$. The solution $\mathbf{u}_1$ is a vector of length d_1 and director $\hat{\mathbf{e}}_1$:

$$U_{10}\hat{\mathbf{e}}_0 = d_1 \hat{\mathbf{e}}_1 \tag{3.2.41}$$

and $\hat{\mathbf{e}}_1$ has a unit norm. Now we apply U_{21} to $\hat{\mathbf{e}}_1$ and obtain a vector of length d_2 and direction $\hat{e}_2$. Finally we can rewrite (3.2.40) as the product of n numbers

$$\mathbf{u}_n = d_n \, d_{n-1} \, \cdots \, d_1 \, \hat{e}_n \quad , \quad \|\hat{e}_n\| = 1 \tag{3.2.42}$$

instead of a product of n matrices. The maximal Lyapunov exponent is then defined as

$$\sigma = \lim_{n \to \infty} \frac{1}{n} \, ln \, \| \, d_1 \, \hat{e}_n \|$$

$$= \lim_{n \to \infty} \frac{1}{n} \sum_{j=1}^{n} ln \, d_n \quad . \tag{3.2.43}$$

We see from the definition of $d_k = \| \, U_{k,k-1} \, \hat{e}_{n-1} \|$ that $ln \, d_k$ is the exponential change of the length of $\hat{e}_0$ during the time interval when the system (3.2.36) moves between the iterates $\mathbf{X}_{k-1}$ and $\mathbf{X}_k$.

Rather than finding just the maximal Lyapunov exponent we can define a Lyapunov exponent for each of the N variables that describe the dynamic system. To do this we note (cf. Benettin, Golgani and Strebyn, 1976) that one can introduce eigenvalues $\lambda_j(n)$ of the matrix

$$\mathbf{A}_n = \left[\mathbf{A}(\mathbf{X}_n) \, \mathbf{A}(\mathbf{X}_{n-1}) \, \cdots \, \mathbf{A}(\mathbf{X}_1) \right]^{1/n} \quad , \tag{3.2.44}$$

where $\mathbf{A}_n$ is defined by (3.2.39) and is the Jacobian matrix of **f**. The Lyapunov exponents are then given by

$$\sigma_j = \; = \lim_{n \to \infty} ln \, | \lambda_j(n) | \quad . \tag{3.2.45}$$

These eigenvalues λ_j are often called the Lyapunov numbers.

Let us consider the example given by Ott (1985) (cf. Figure 3.2.10). For a two-dimensional map, the Lyapunov numbers are given by λ_1 and λ_2 and are interpreted as the average principle stretching factors for a very small initial circular area of radius $\varepsilon(0)$. More formally we can write

$$\lambda_j = \lim_{n \to \infty} \Bigg\{ \text{magnitude of the } j^{th} \text{ eigenvaues of}$$

$$\left[\mathbf{A}(X_n, Y_n) \, \mathbf{A}(X_{n-1}, Y_{n-1}) \, \cdots \, \mathbf{A}(X_1, Y_1) \right]^{1/n} \Bigg\} \quad , \tag{3.2.46}$$

where $\mathbf{A}(X, Y)$ is the Jacobian matrix of the map:

150

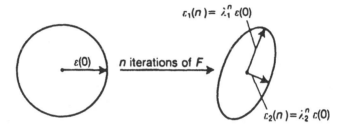

$$c_1(n) = \lambda_1^n \, \varepsilon(0)$$

$\varepsilon(0)$

n iterations of F

$$c_2(n) = \lambda_2^n \, c(0)$$

Figure 3.2.10. Lyapunov exponents define the average stretching or contraction of trajectories in characteristic directions. Here we show the effects of
applying a two-dimensional mapping to circles of initial conditions. A
sufficiently small circle of radius ε is transformed after n iterations into
an ellipse with major radius $\lambda_1^n \varepsilon$ and minor radius $\lambda_2^n \varepsilon$, where λ_1 and
λ_2 are the Lyapunov exponents for $n \to \infty$.

$$A(X,Y) = \begin{bmatrix} \dfrac{\partial f_1(X,Y)}{\partial X} & \dfrac{\partial f_1(X,Y)}{\partial Y} \\ \dfrac{\partial f_2(X,Y)}{\partial X} & \dfrac{\partial f_2(X,Y)}{\partial Y} \end{bmatrix} . \qquad (3.2.47)$$

The functions f_1 and f_2 are the components of the mapping vector $\mathbf{f}$ in (3.2.36); and, of course, $(X_1 Y_1)$, $\cdots$, (X_n, Y_n) is a sequence generated by the map. Then the Lyapunov numbers specify the average stretching rate of nearby points. If the map is to be chaotic, for $\lambda_1 > \lambda_2$ say, then λ_1 must be greater than unity, so that the distance between almost nearby points increases in successive iterations. If the map is area contracting then $\lambda_1 \lambda_2 < 1$, the distance between almost nearby points decreases in successive iterations; if it is area preserving then $\lambda_1 \lambda_2 = 1$ and the distance remains unchanged.

3.3 Measures of Strange Attractors

In broad outline we have attempted to give some indications of how simple non-linear dynamic equations can give rise to a rich variety of dynamic behaviors. In particular we have, in large part, focused on the phenomenon of chaos described from the point of view of mathematics and modeling. Some effort has been made to put these discussions in a biomedical context, but little or no effort was made to relate these results to actual data sets. Thus the techniques may not appear to be as useful as they could be to the experimentalist who observes large variations in his/her data and wonders if the observed fluctuations are chaos or noise. In most biomedical phenomena there is no reliable dynamical model describing the behavior of the system, so the investigator must use the data directly to distinguish between the two; there is no guide telling what the appropriate parameters are that might be varied. As we mentioned earlier, a traditional method for determining the dynamical content of a time series is to construct the power spectrum for the process by taking the Fourier transform of the autocorrelation function, or equivalently by taking the Fourier transform of the time series itself and forming its absolute square [cf. (3.1.16)].

The autocorrelation function provides a way to use the data at one time to determine the influence of the process on itself at a latter time. It is a measure of the relation of the value of a random process at one instant of time, $X(t)$ say, to the value at another instant τ seconds later, $X(t + \tau)$. If we have a data record extending continuously over the time interval $(-T/2, T/2)$, then the autocorrelation function can be defined as

$$C_{xx}(\tau) \equiv \lim_{T \to \infty} \frac{1}{T} \int_{-T/2}^{T/2} X(t)X(t+\tau)\, dt \quad . \tag{3.3.1}$$

Note that for a finite sample length, i.e., for T finite, the integral defines an *estimate* for the autocorrelation function $C_{xx}(\tau,T)$ so that $C_{xx}(\tau) = \lim_{T \to \infty} C_{xx}(\tau,T)$. In Figure 3.3.1 a sample history of $X(t)$ is given along with its displaced time trace $X(t+\tau)$. The point by point product of these two series is given in (3.3.1) and then the average over the time interval $(-T/2, T/2)$ is taken. A sine wave, or any other harmonic deterministic data set, would have an autocorrelation function which persists over all time displacements. Thus the autocorrelation function can provide a measure of deterministic data embedded in a random background.

Similar comments apply when the data set is discrete rather than continuous, as it would be for the mappings in Section 3.2. In the discrete case we denote the interval between samples as $\Delta(=T/N)$ for N equally spaced intervals and r as the lag or delay number so that the estimated autocorrelation function is

$$C_{xx}(r\Delta,N) = \frac{1}{N-r} \sum_{j=1}^{N-r} X_j X_{j+r} \, , \; r = 0, 1, \cdots, m \tag{3.3.2}$$

and m is the maximum lag number. Note that $C_{xx}(r\Delta,N)$ is analogous to the estimate of the continuum autocorrelation function and becomes the true autocorrelation function in the limit $N \to \infty$. These considerations have been discussed at great length by Wiener (1949) in his classic book on time series analysis, and is still recommended today as a text from which to capture a master's style of investigation.

The frequency content is extracted from the time series using the autocorrelation function by applying a filter in the form of a Fourier transform. This yield the power spectral density

$$S_{xx}(\omega) = \frac{1}{\pi} \int_{-\infty}^{\infty} e^{-i\omega t} C_{xx}(t)\, dt \tag{3.3.3}$$

of the time series $X(t)$. Equation (3.3.3) relates the autocorrelation function to the power spectral density and is known as the *Weiner-Khinchine* relation in agreement with (3.1.15). One example of its use is provided in Figure 3.3.2a where the exponential form of the autocorrelation function $C_{xx}(t) = e^{-t/\tau_c}$ used in Figure 3.3.2b yields a frequency spectrum of the Cauchy form

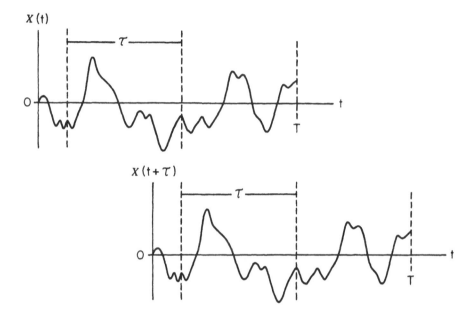

Figure 3.3.1. The time trace of a random function $X(t)$ versus time t is shown in the upper curve. The lower curve is the same time trace displaced by a time interval τ. The product of these two functions when averaged yield an estimate of the autocorrelation function $C_{xx}(\tau, T)$.

154

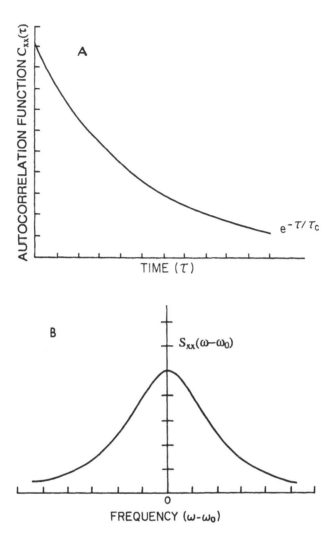

Figure 3.3.2. (a) The autocorrelation function $C_{xx}(\tau)$ for the typical time traces depicted in Figure 3.3.1 assuming the fluctuations are exponentially correlated in time $[\exp(-\tau/\tau_c)]$. The constant τ_c is the time required for $C_{xx}(\tau)$ to decrease by a factor $1/e$, this is the decorrelation time. (b) The power spectral density $S_{xx}(\omega)$ is graphed as a function of frequency for the exponential correlation function with a central frequency ω_0.

$$S_{xx}(\omega) = \frac{1}{\pi} \frac{\tau_c}{1 + \omega^2 \tau_c^2} \ . \tag{3.3.4}$$

At high frequencies the spectrum (3.3.4) is seen to fall-off as ω^{-2}. Basar (1980), among others, has applied these techniques to the analysis of many medical phenomena including the interpretation of electrical signals from the brain.

The electrical activity of the brain measured at various points on the scalp is well known to be quite erratic. It was the dream of the mathematician Norbert Wiener (1964) that the methods of *harmonic decomposition* would force the brain to yield up its secrets as a generalized control system. In this early approach the aperiodic signal captured in the EEG time series is assumed to consist of a superposition of independent frequency modes. This assumption enabled the investigator to interpret the harmonic content of the EEG signal using the above Fourier methods. This view was partially reinforced by the work on evoked potentials, discussed in Chapter 4, where a clear pattern in the EGG signal could be reproduced with specific external stimulations such as auditory tones. In Figure 3.3.3 a typical set of averaged evoked potentials for a sleeping cat is depicted. The large initial bump is produced by auditory stimulation in the form of a step function. The corresponding PSD is depicted in Figure 3.3.4. Here again we have an inverse power law in frequency for high frequency. In fact, it is very close to the ω^{-2} asymptotic shape of the Cauchy PSD.

As we mentioned, a periodic signal in the data will show sharp peaks in the spectrum corresponding to the fundamental frequency and its higher harmonics [cf. Section 3.1(b)]. On the other hand the spectrum corresponding to aperiodic variations in the time series will be broadband in frequency with no discernible structure. In themselves spectral techniques have no way of discriminating between chaos and noise and are therefore of little value in determining the *source* of the fluctuations in a data set. They were in fact very useful, as shown in Section 3.1(b), in establishing the *similarities* between stochastic processes and chaos defined as the sensitive dependence on initial conditions in a dynamic process.

One way in which some investigators have proceeded in discriminating between chaos and noise is to visually examine time series for period doublings. This is a somewhat risky business, however, and may lead to misinterpretations of data sets. Also, period doubling is only one of the possible routes to chaos in dynamic systems. For

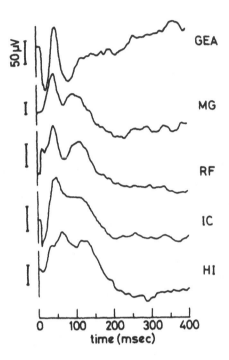

Figure 3.3.3. A typical set of simultaneously recorded and selectively averaged evoked potentials in different brain nuclei of chronically implanted cats, elicited during the slow wave sleep stage by an auditory stimulation in the form of step function. Direct computer-plottings. Negativity upwards (after Basar, Gonder, Ozesmi and Ungar, 1975).

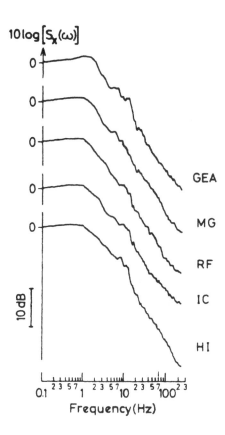

Figure 3.3.4. Mean value curves of the power spectral density functions obtained from
16 experiments during the slow wave sleep stage. Direct computer-
plottings. Along the abscissa is the frequency in logarithmic scale, along
the ordinate the power spectral density, $S_x(\omega)$, in such a way that the
power at 0 Hz is equal to 1 (or 10 log 1 = 0) (after Basar et al., 1975).

example considerable attention is again being focused on the possible dynamical mechanisms underlying cardiac electrical disturbances. The abrupt onset of an arrhythmia appears to represent a bifurcation from the stable, physiological steady state of normal sines rhythm to one involving different frequency modes. Perhaps the most compelling evidence for the relevance of nonlinear analysis to these perturbations comes from recent reports of period-doubling phenomena during a variety of induced and spontaneous arrhythmias (see Section 4.3).

The major question guiding future investigations in this case is whether nonlinear models will provide new understanding of the mechanisms of sudden cardiac death. The most important fatal arrhythmia is ventricular fibrillation, characterized by rapid, apparently erratic oscillations of the electrocardiogram. The notion that ventricular fibrillation represents a form of cardiac chaos has been at large for many years. The term ''chaotic'' to describe this arrhythmia was first used in a colloquial sense by investigators and clinicians observing the seemingly random oscillations of the electrocardiogram which were associated with ineffective, uncoordinated twitching of the dying heart muscle. This generic use of the term ''chaos'' to describe fibrillation underwent an important evolution in 1964 when Moe, Rheinboldt and Abildskov proposed a model of atrial fibrillation as a turbulent cascade of large waves into small eddies and smaller wavelets, etc. The concept that ventricular fibrillation represent a similar type of ''completely chaotic, turbulent'' process was advanced most recently by Smith and Cohen (1984). Furthermore, based on previous evidence for 2:1 alternation in the ECG waveform preceding the onset of fibrillation, Smith and Cohen raised the provocative notion that fibrillation of the heart might follow the subharmonic bifurcation route to chaos. This speculation-linking recent nonlinear models of chaotic behavior to the understanding of sudden cardiac death has occasioned considerable interest.

One approach to testing this hypothesis is by means of spectral analysis of fibrillatory waveforms. If fibrillation is a homogeneous turbulent process then it should be associated with a broadband spectrum with appropriate scaling characteristics. However, the finding presented by Goldberger et al. (1986) in concert with multiple previous spectral and autocorrelation analyses (Nygards and Hulting, 1977; Angelakos and Shephard, 1957) as well as recent electrophysiologic mapping data (Ideker, Klein and Harrison, 1981; Worley, Swain, and Colavita, 1985) suggest the need to reassess this concept of fibrillation as cardiac chaos. Furthermore, spectral analysis of electrocardiographic data may have more general implications for modeling transitions from physiological stability to pathological oscillatory behavior in a wide variety of other life-threatening conditions, (Goldberger and West, 1987c).

The relatively narrow-band spectrum of fibrillatory signals contrast with the spectrum of the normal ventricular depolarization (QRS) waveform which in man and animals shows a wide band of frequencies (0 to > 300 Hz) with $1/f$-like scaling (i.e. power spectral density at frequency f is equal to $1/f^\alpha$ where α is a positive number). As discussed in Section 2.4 we recently related the power-law scaling that characterizes the spectrum of the normal QRS waveform to the underlying fractal geometry of the branching His-Purkinje system. Furthermore, a broadband inverse power-law spectrum has also been identified by analysis of interbeat intervals variations in a group of healthy subjects, indicating that normal sinus rhythm is not a strictly periodic state. Important phasic changes in heart rate associated with respiration and other physiologic control systems account for only some of the variability in heartbeat interval dynamics; overall, the spectrum in healthy subjects includes a much wider band of frequencies with $1/f$ —like scaling. This behavior is also observed in the EEG time series data.

It has been suggested that fractal processes associated with scaled, broadband spectra are "information-rich." Periodic states, in contrast, reflect narrow-band spectra and are defined by monotonous, repetitive sequences, depleted of information content. In Figure 3.3.5 we depict the spectrum of the time series $X(t)$ obtained from the funnel attractor solution of the equation set (3.1.19)-(3.1.21). The attractor itself is shown in Figure 3.1.20. We see that the spectrum is broad band as was that of the Lorenz attractor (cf. Figure 3.1.18), with a number of relatively sharp spikes. These spikes are manifestations of a strong periodic components in the dynamics of the funnel attractor. Thus the dynamics could easily be interpreted in terms of a number of harmonic components in a noisy background, but this would be an error. One way to distinguish between these two interpretations is by means of the information dimension of the time series. The dimension decreases as a system undergoes a transition from chaotic to periodic dynamics. The transition from healthy function to disease implies an analogous loss of physiological information and is consistent with a transition from a wide-band to a narrow-band spectrum. The dominance of relatively low-frequency periodic oscillations might be anticipated as a hallmark of the dynamics of many types of severe pathophysiologic disturbances. As pointed out earlier, such periodicities have already been documented in

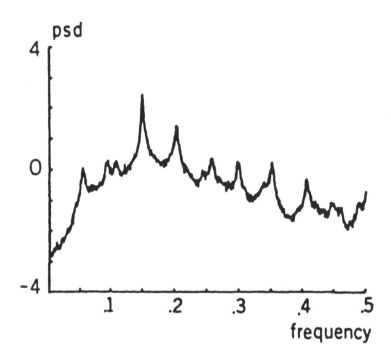

Figure 3.3.5. The power spectral density for the $X(t)$ time series for the "funnel" depicted in Figure 3.1.20.

many advanced clinical settings, including Cheyne-Stokes breathing patterns in heart failure, leukemic cell production, sinusoidal heart rate oscillations in fetal distress syndromes, and the "swinging heart" phenomenon in cardiac tamponade. The highly periodic electrical fibrillatory activity of the heart, which is associated with ineffective mechanical contraction and sudden death, is perhaps the most dramatic example of this kind of abnormal spectral periodicity. More subtle alterations in the spectral features of cardiovascular function have also been described, including decreased high frequency QRS potentials in some cases of chronic myocardial infraction in contrast to increased high frequency potentials in healthy subjects in the "supraphysiologic" state of exercise. Ventricular fibrillation may serve, therefore, as a general model for transitions from broadband stability to certain types of pathological periodicities in other physiological disturbances.

Thus we conclude that more systematic methods for distinguishing between chaos and noise are desirable and necessary. We turn to some of those methods now.

(a)   **Correlational dimension**

In the preceding discussion we presented the standard example of a correlation function having an exponential form. Such a correlation function could describe a random time series having a memory or correlation time τ_c. It could not describe a dynamical system having an asymptotic stationary or periodic state. Similarly it could not describe a nonlinear dissipative dynamical system that has a chaotic attractor. Grassberger and Procaccia (1983) developed a correlational technique by which one can exclude various choices for the kind of attractor on which the dynamics for a given data set exists. They wanted to be able to say that the attractor for the data set is not multiply periodic, or that the irregularities are not due to external noise, etc. As we have just seen Fourier analysis would tell us if the attractor were multiply periodic, but not the source of the fluctuations. They proposed a measure obtained by considering correlations between points of a time series taken from a trajectory on the attractor after the initial transients have died away.

Consider the set $\{X_j, j = 1, 2, \cdots, M\}$ of points on the attractor taken from a vector time series $X(t)$, i.e., we take $X_j \equiv X(t + j\tau)$ where τ is a fixed time interval between successive measurements. The vector time series $X(t)$ could be the three components of the Lorenz model, $X(t) \equiv \{X(t), Y(t), Z(t)\}$ or those of the Rössler model or even the two components of the Hénon model. In the latter case the "time" series would already be discrete and the set of M points could be all the iterates of the map or it could be a selected subset of the generated points. If the attractor is chaotic then since nearby trajectories exponentially separate in time, we expect that most pairs of points $\mathbf{X}_j$, $\mathbf{X}_k$ $j \neq k$ will be dynamically uncorrelated. Even though these points may appear to be essentially random, they do all lie on the same attractor and therefore are correlated in phase space. Grassberger and Procaccia (1983) introduced the correlation integral $C(r)$ defined by

$$C(r) \equiv \lim_{M \to \infty} \frac{1}{M(M-1)} \sum_{i,j=1}^{M} \Theta \left(r - |\mathbf{X}_i - \mathbf{X}_j| \right)$$

$$\equiv \int_0^r d^E r' \, c(\mathbf{r}') \qquad (3.3.5)$$

where $\Theta(x)$ is the Heaviside function, $=0$ if $x \leq 0$ and $=1$ if $x > 0$, and $c(\mathbf{r}')$ is the traditional correlation function in E-Euclidian dimensions:

$$c(\mathbf{r}) = \lim_{M \to \infty} \frac{1}{M(M-1)} \sum_{i,j=1, i \neq j}^{M} \delta^E (\mathbf{X}_i - \mathbf{X}_j - \mathbf{r}) \ . \qquad (3.3.6)$$

The virtue of the integral function is that for a chaotic or strange attractor the correlational integral has the power-law form

$$C(r) \sim r^\nu \qquad (3.3.7)$$

and moreover, the "correlation exponent" ν is closely related to the fractal dimension d and the information dimension σ of the attractor. They argue that the correlation exponent is a useful measure of the local properties of the attractor whereas the fractal dimension is a purely geometric measure and is rather insensitive to the local dynamic behavior of the trajectories on the attractor. The information dimension is somewhat sensitive to the local behavior of the trajectories and is a lower bound on the Hausdorff dimension. In fact they observe that in general one has

$$\nu \leq \sigma \leq d \ . \qquad (3.3.8)$$

Thus if the correlation integral obtained from an experimental data set has the power-law form (3.3.7) with $\nu < E$, they argue that one knows that the data set arises from deterministic chaos rather than random noise, because noise will result in $C(r) \sim r^E$ for a constant correlation function over the distance r. Note that for periodic sequences $\nu = 1$; for random sequences it should equal the embedding dimension, while for chaotic sequences it is finite and non-integer.

Grassberger and Procassia establish (3.3.7) by the following argument: If the attractor is a fractal, then the number of hypercubes of edge length r needed to cover it $N(r)$ is

$$N(t) \sim \frac{1}{r^d} \tag{3.3.9}$$

(cf. Chapter 2). The number of points from the data set which are in the jth nonempty cube is denoted n_j so that

$$C(r) \sim \frac{1}{M^2} \sum_{j=1}^{N(r)} n_j^2 = \frac{N(r)}{M^2} <n^2> \tag{3.3.10}$$

up to $O(1)$, and the angular brackets denote an average over all occupied cells. By the Schwartz inequality $(<n^2> \geq <n>^2)$:

$$C(r) \geq \frac{N(r)}{M^2} <n>^2 = \frac{1}{M^2 N(r)} \left[\sum_{j=1}^{N(r)} n_j \right]^2 \tag{3.3.11}$$

but

$$\sum_{j=1}^{N(r)} n_j = M \tag{3.3.12}$$

so that using (3.3.9)

$$C(r) \geq \frac{1}{N(r)} = r^d \quad . \tag{3.3.13}$$

Thus comparing (3.3.13) with (3.3.7) they obtain the inequality

$$\nu \leq d \quad , \tag{3.3.14}$$

so that the correlation dimension is less than or equal to the fractal dimension.

Grassberger and Procaccia also point out that one of the main advantages of the correlation dimension ν is the ease with which it can be measured. In particular it can be measured more easily than either σ or d for cases when the fractal dimension is large (≥ 3). Just as they anticipated, the measure ν has proven to be most useful in experimental situations, where typically high dimensional systems exist. However, we point out in Section 3.3c that calculating the fractal dimension in this way does not establish that the erratic time series is generated by a chaotic attractor. It only proves that the time series is fractal.

To test their ideas they studied the behavior of a number of simple models for which the fractal dimension is known. In Figure 3.3.6 we display three of the many calculations they did. In each case the logarithm of the correlation integral $[ln\,C(r)]$ is plotted as a function of the logarithm of a dimensionless length $(ln\ r)$ which according to the power-law relation (3.3.7) should yield a straight line of positive slope. The slope of the line is the correlational dimension ν. We see from these examples that the technique successfully predicts the correlational behavior for both chaotic mappings and differential equations having solutions on chaotic attractors.

(b)   Attractor reconstruction from data

More often than not the biomedical experimentalist does not have the luxury of a mathematical model to guide the measurement process. What is usually available are a few partial theories, securely based on assumptions often made more for convenience than for reality, and a great deal of phenomenology. Therefore in a system known to depend on a number of independent variables it is not clear how many kinds of measurements one should make. In fact it is often unrealistically difficult to take more than the measurement of a single degree of freedom. What then can one say about a complex system given this single time series? Such questions are relevant, for example, in determining what can be learned about the functioning of the brain using EEG time series; in what can be learned about the dynamics of epidemics using only the number of people infected with a disease; in what can be learned about the excitability of single neurons from the time series of post synaptic pulses; in what can be learned about biochemical reactions by monitoring a single chemical species and so on. It turns out that quite a lot can be learned using methods developed in nonlinear dynamics. In particular a method has been devised that enables one to reconstruct a multidimensional attractor from the time series of a single observable. The application of this technique to a number of data sets will be reviewed in the next chapter, but for the moment we concentrate on the exposition of the underlying theory.

Packard, Crutchfield, Farmer and Shaw (1980) who constituted the nucleus of the *Dynamic Systems Collective* at the University of California, Santa Cruz in the late 70's and early 80's, were the first investigators to demonstrate how one reconstructs a chaotic attractor from an actual data set. They used the time series generated by one coordinate of the three-dimensional chaotic dynamical system studied by Rössler (1978), i.e.,

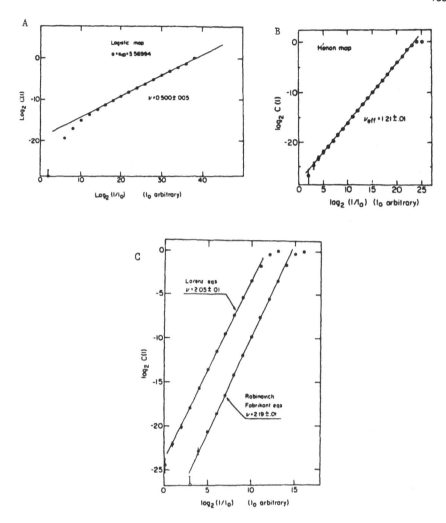

Figure 3.3.6.   (a) The correlation integral for the logistic map (3.2.11) at the infinite
bifurcation point $\mu = \mu_\infty = 3.699 \cdots$ The starting point was $Y_0 = 1/2$, the
number of points was $N = 3 \times 10^4$. (b) Correlation integral for the Henon
map (3.2.29) and (3.2.30) with $c = 1.4, \beta = 0.01$ and $N = 1.5 \times 10^4$. (c)
Correlation integrals for the Lorenz equations (3.1.9)-(3.1.11) (dots); for
the Rabinovich-Fabricant equation (open circles).   In both cases
$N = 1.5 \times 10^4$ and $\tau = 0.25$. (From Grassberger and Procaccia, 1985.)
(From Grassburger and Procaccia, 1983a.)

(3.1.19)-(3.1.21) with the parameter values $a = 0.2$, $b = 0.4$ and $c = 5.7$. The reconstruction method is based on the hueristic idea that for such a three-dimensional system, any three "independent" time varying quantities are sufficient to specify the state of the system. The three dynamic coordinates $X(t)$, $Y(t)$ and $Z(t)$ are only one of the many possible choices. They conjectured that; "any such sets of three independent quantities which uniquely and smoothly label the states of the attractor are diffeomorphically equivalent." In English this means that an actual dynamic system does not know of the particular representation chosen by us, and that any other representation containing the same dynamic information is just as good. Thus, an experimentalist sampling the values of a single coordinate need not find the "one" representation favored by nature, since this "one" does not in all probability exist.

Packard et al. (1980) playing the role of experimentalists sampled the $X(t)$ coordinate of the Rössler attractor. They then noted a number of possible alternatives to the phase space coordinates (x, y, z) that could give a faithful representation of the dynamics using the time series they had obtained. One possible set was the $X(t)$ time series itself plus two replicas of it displaced in time by τ and 2τ, i.e. $X(t)$, $X(t+\tau)$ and $X(t+2\tau)$. Note that implicit in this choice is the idea that $X(t)$ is so strongly coupled to the other degrees of freedom that it contains dynamic information about these coordinates as well as itself. A second representation set is obtained by making the time interval τ an infinitesimal, so that by taking differences between the variables we obtain $X(t)$, $\dot{X}(t)$ and $\ddot{X}(t)$.

Figure 3.1.20d shows a projection of the Rössler chaotic attractor on the (x, y) plane. Figure 3.3.7 depicts the reconstruction of that attractor from the sampled $X(t)$ time series in the $(x, \dot{x})$ plane. It is clear that the two attractors are not identical, but it is just as clear that the reconstructed one retains the topological characteristics and geometrical form of the experimental attractor. One quantitative measure of the equivalence of the experimental and reconstructed attractors is the Lyapunov exponent associated with each one. This exponent can be determined by constructing a *return map* for each of the attractors and then applying the relation (3.2.31).

A return map is obtained by constructing a Poincaré surface of section. In this example of an attractor projected onto a two-dimensional plane, the Poincaré surface of section is the intersection of the attractor with a line transverse to the attractor. We indicate this by the dashed line in Figure 3.3.7 and the measured data are the sequence of

A

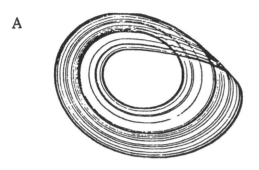

B

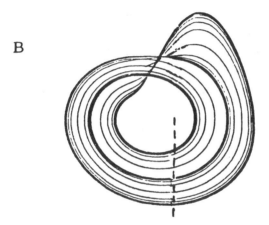

Figure 3.3.7. A two-dimensional projection of the Rossler chaotic attractor (a) is compared with the reconstruction in the $(\dot{x}, x)$ plane of the attractor (b) from
the time series $x(t)$. The dashed line indicates the Poincaré surface of
section for this attractor (from Packard et al., 1980).

values $\{X_n\}$ denoting the crossing of the line by the attractor in the positive direction. These data are used to construct a next amplitude plot in which each amplitude X_{n+1} is plotted as a function of the preceding amplitude X_n. It is possible for such a plot to yield anything from a random spray of points to a well defined curve. If in fact we find a curve with a definite structure then it may be possible to construct a return map for the attractor. For example, the oscillating chemical reaction of Belousov and Zhabotinskii was shown by Simoyi, Wolf, and Swinney (1980) to be describable by such a one-dimensional map. In Figure 3.3.8 we indicate the return map constructed from the experimental data of Simoyi et al. (1980), also Figure 3.1.19 for the Lorenz attractor.

Simoyi et al. (1982) point out that there are 25 or so distinct chemicals in the Belousov-Zhabotinskii reaction, many more than can be reliably monitored. Therefore there is no way to construct the twenty-five dimensional phase space $X(t)$ $= \{X_1(t), X_2(t), \cdots X_{25}(t)\}$ from the experimental data. Instead they use the embedding theorems of Whitney (1936) and Takens (1981) to justify the monitoring of a single chemical species, in this case the concentration of the bromide ion, for use in constructing an m-dimensional phase portrait of the attractor $\{X(t), X(t+\tau), \cdots X[t+(m-1)\tau]\}$ for sufficiently large m and for almost any time delay τ. They find that for their experimental data $m=3$ is adequate and the resulting one-dimensional map (cf. Figure 3.3.8) provided the first example of a physical system with many degrees of freedom that can be so modeled in detail.

Let us now recap the technique. We assume that the system of interest, can be described by m variables, where m is large but *unknown*, so that at any instant of time there is a point $X(t) = [X_1(t), X_2(t), \cdots, X_m(t)]$ in an m-dimensional phase space that completely characterizes the system. This point moves around as the system evolves, in some cases approaching a fixed point or limit cycle asymptotically in time. In other cases the motion appears to be purely random and one must distinguish between a system confined to a chaotic attractor and one driven by noise. In experiments, one often only records the output of a single detector, which selects one of the N components of the system for monitoring. In general the experimentalist does not know the size of the phase space since the important dynamic variables are usually not known and therefore he/she must extract as much information as possible from the single time series available, $X_1(t)$ say. For sufficiently long times τ one uses the embedding theorem to construct the sequence of displaced time series $\{X_1(t), X_1(t+\tau), \ldots, X_1[t+(m-1)\tau]\}$. This set of variables has been shown to have the same amount of information as the

169

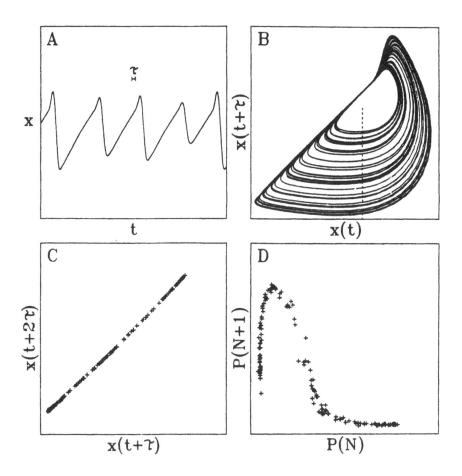

Figure 3.3.8. Attractor from a chemical oscillator. (a) The time series $X(t)$ is the bromide ion concentration in a Belousov-Zhabatinskii reaction. A time interval τ is indicated. (b) Plot of $X(t)$ versus $X(t+\tau)$. Dotted line indicates a cut through the attractor. (c) Cross section of attractor along cut. (d) Poincaré return map of cut, $P(N+1)$ is the position the trajectory crosses the dotted line as a function of the crossing position on the previous turn around the attractor (from Roux and Swinney, 1981).

d-dimensional phase point provided that $m \geq 2d + 1$. Thus, as time goes to infinity, we can build from the experimental data a one-dimensional phase space $X_1(t)$, a two-dimensional phase space with axes $\{X_1(t), X_1(t+\tau)\}$, a three-dimensional phase space with axes $\{X_1(t), X_1(t+\tau), X_1(t+2\tau)\}$, and so on. The condition on the embedding dimension m, i.e. $m \geq 2d + 1$, is often overly restrictive and the reconstructed attractor does not require m to be so large.

Grassberger and Procaccia (1983, 1985) extended their original method, being inspired by the work of Packard et al. (1980) and Takens (1981), to the embedding procedure just described. Instead of using the $\mathbf{X}_j$ data set discussed previously, they employ the m-dimensional vector

$$\xi(t_j) = \left\{ X_1(t_j), X_1(t_j + \tau), \ldots, X_1\left[t_j + (m-1)\tau\right] \right\} \tag{3.3.15}$$

from m-copies of the original time series $X_1(t)$. The m-dimensional correlation integral is

$$C_m(r) = \lim_{M \to \infty} \frac{1}{M(M-1)} \sum_{l,k=1}^{M} \Theta\left(r - |\xi(t_l) - \xi(t_k)|\right) \tag{3.3.16}$$

which for a chaotic (fractal) time series again has the power-law form

$$C_m(r) \sim r^{\nu_m} \tag{3.3.17}$$

where

$$\lim_{m \to \infty} \nu_m = \nu \tag{3.3.18}$$

and ν is again the correlation dimension. In Figure 3.3.6 the results for the Lorenz model with $m=3$ is depicted where $X_1(t) \equiv X(t)$; the power-law is still satisfactory being in essential agreement with the earlier result.

(c)   **Chaotic attractors and false alarms**

The correlational integral of Grassberger and Procaccia was devised to determine the dimensionality of an attractor from time series data, assuming that such an attractor does in fact exist. It has been pointed out by Osborne and and Provenzale (1988) that this has not been how the correlation dimension has been used in the analysis of experimental data sets. The procedure has been to apply the embedding procedure to a measured time series from a dissipative system, and if the evaluation of (3.3.16) yields a finite value for the correlation dimension, then the system is thought to be describable by deterministic dynamics. Further, if the value of ν is low and noninteger then the dynamics are argued to be governed by a strange attractor and are therefore chaotic. This logical fallacy has been particularly apparent in the analysis of geophysical data sets [see e.g. Nicolis and Nicolis (1984) and Fraedrich (1986)].

One reason for the misapplication of the correlation dimension is the recognition that for a stochastic process the correlation integral diverges as a power law with the power law index ν_m being given by the embedding dimension. This situation arises because a stochastic or random time series is believed to completely fill the available volume whereas a chaotic time series is restricted to an attractor of finite dimension $d \geq \nu$ lower than the embedding dimension m as m becomes large. This widely held belief is based on the example of Gaussian white noise for the random time series, but has in fact been shown by a number of investigators not to be a general result [Theiler (1986); Osborne and Provenzale (1988)]. The crux of the matter is that the Grassberger-Procaccia measure determines if the time series is fractal or not, but not the cause of its being fractal. While it is true that a low-dimensional chaotic attractor will generate a fractal time series, so too will other multiple-scale processes. For example a scalar wave scattered from a fractal surface will itself become a fractal times series [Berry (1979)], or the cardiac pulse traversing the fractal His-Purkinje condition system results in a fractal times series [Goldberger, et al. (1985)] as we discussed in Chapter 2.

Osborne and Provenzale (1988) calculate a finite and well defined value for the correlation dimension for a class of random noises with inverse power-law spectra. The time series they consider is given by the discrete Fourier representation

$$X(t_j) = \sum_{l=1}^{M/2} \left[S(\omega_l) \Delta \omega_l \right]^{1/2} \cos(\omega_l t_j + \phi_l) ; \quad j=1, 2 \ldots, M , \qquad (3.3.19)$$

where $\omega_l = 2\pi l / M \Delta t$, Δt is the sampling interval and M is the number of data points in the time series. The time series $X(t_j)$ is random if the set of phases $\{\phi_l\}$ consist of random variables uniformly distributed on the interval $(0, 2\pi)$. In this case $S(\omega_l)$ is the power spectrum of the time series denoting the way in which energy is distributed over the frequencies contributing to the series.

As we discussed in Chapter 2 a fractal process is free of a characteristic time scale and is expected to have an inverse power law spectrum [see also Voss (1988)]. Thus, Osborne and Provenzale investigated the properties of the times series (3.3.19) with

$$S(\omega_l) = \frac{C}{\omega_l^{\alpha}} \qquad (3.3.20)$$

where $C > 0$ is chosen to yield a unit variance for the times series and $\alpha > 0$. Such time series are said to be "colored" noise and have generated a great deal of interest recently in the physical sciences [Moss and McClintoch (1989)].

Osborne and Provenzale calculated $\mathbf{X}(t) = \{X_1(t), X_2(t), \ldots, X_m(t)\}$ for fifteen different values of the embedding dimension $m = 1, 2, \ldots 15$ for specific values of α. The correlation function (3.3.16) is then calculated for each value of m and $\ln C_m(r)$ is graphed versus $\ln r$ in Figure 3.3.9. The slope of these curves yields ν_m from (3.3.17)

$$\ln C_m(r) = \nu_m \ln r + \text{constant} . \qquad (3.3.21)$$

This value of ν_m is then plotted versus the embedding dimension in the associated figure. If the values of ν_m saturate for increasing m, then from (3.3.18) we obtain the value of the correlation dimension. One would have expected that since $\mathbf{X}(t)$ is a stochastic process that no saturation value exists, but this is seen not to be the case as α increases.

In Figure 3.3.9a they show fifteen correlation functions $C_m(r)$ for $m = 1, 2, \ldots 15$ with $\alpha = 1.0$ in (3.3.20). This corresponds to a white noise spectrum. The straight line region of the figure yields ν_m from (3.3.21). Figure 3.3.9b shows ν_m versus m, where no saturation is evident as one would have expected. In Figure 3.3.10a the fifteen values of the correlation function are depicted for $\alpha = 1.75$. Again scaling is seen to be present from the straight line region of the graph, and as shown in Figure 3.3.10b the values of ν_m do saturate for large m to the value $\nu \cong 2.66$. As they point out: "This traditionally unexpected result thus implies that a finite value for the correlation dimension ν may be found even for non-deterministic, random signals." Thus by repeating this analysis for a number of values α they find a quantitative relation between ν and α. This relation $\nu(\alpha)$ is shown in Figure 3.3.11, where we see that for $\alpha \geq 3$ the correlation function saturates at a value of unity. From these results it is clear that for white noise there is no correlation dimension, but that is *not* true in general for random processes with inverse power-law spectra.

As we discussed in Chapter 2 a fractal stochastic process is self-affine so that if we consider an increment of $X(t)$:

$$\Delta X(\tau) = X(t + \tau) - X(t) . \qquad (3.3.22)$$

and scale the time interval τ by a constant Γ

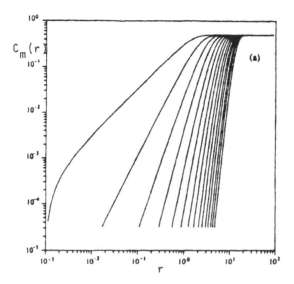

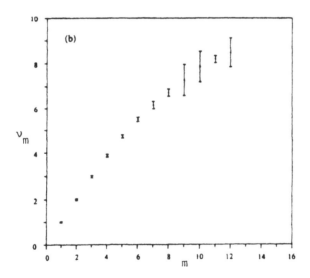

Figure 3.3.9. (a) the fifteen correlation functions $C_m(r)$ for a spectral exponent $\alpha = 1.0$, and (b) the correlation dimension v_m versus the embedding dimension m for this case. No saturation is evident in this case.

174

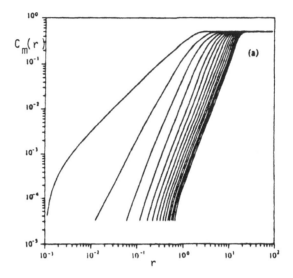

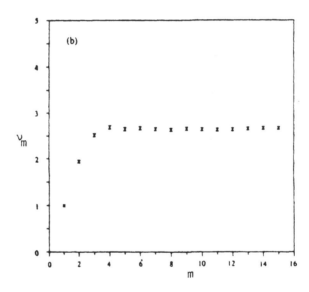

Figure 3.3.10.   (a) the fifteen correlation functions $C_m(r)$ for $\alpha = 1.75$, and (b) the
dimension v_m versus m. The correlation dimension saturates at a value
$v \cong 2.66$.

175

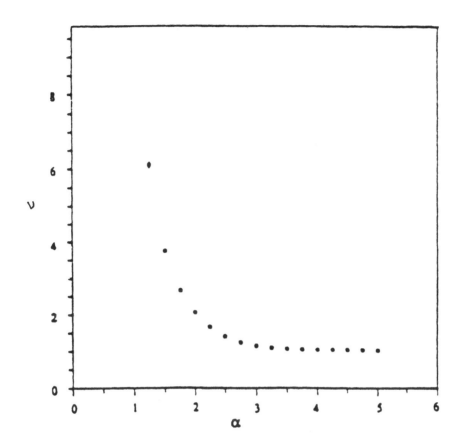

Figure 3.3.11. The correlation dimension ν versus the spectral exponent α. The correlation dimension turns out to be a well defined, monotonically decreasing function ν(α) of the spectral exponent α for this class of random noises.

$$\Delta X (\Gamma\tau) = \Gamma^H \Delta X (\tau) \qquad\qquad (3.3.23)$$

where H is the scaling exponent, $0 < H \le 1$. Now if we generate a self-similar trajectory from the time series (3.3.19) in an m-dimensional phase space, each component has the same scaling exponent H. The fractal dimension of the trajectory generated by the colored noise is then given by Mandelbrot (1977),

$$d = \min \{1/H, m\} \ . \qquad\qquad (3.3.24)$$

Thus for $0 < H < 1$ the trajectory is a fractal curve since its fractal dimension strictly exceeds it topological dimension $D_T = 1$.

Osborne and Provenzale numerically verify the relation (3.2.24) for the colored noise time series. Using the scaling relation (3.2.23) they evaluate the average of the absolute value of the increment in the process $X(t)$:

$$\langle |\Delta X (\Gamma\tau)| \rangle \ \Gamma^H \langle |\Delta X (\tau)| \rangle \ . \qquad\qquad (3.3.25)$$

The average is taken over the fifteen realizations of the stochastic process used earlier as well as over time. If in fact the process is self-affine then a plot of $ln < |\Delta X (\Gamma\tau)| >$ versus $ln \Gamma$ should be a straight line with slope H. In Figure 3.3.12 is shown three straight line curves corresponding to $\alpha = 1.0$, 1.75 and 2.75 with the slope values of $H \cong 0.1$, 0.39 and 0.84 respectively. The fractal dimensions $d = 1/H$ in these three cases are $d \cong 10$, 2.56 and 1.19, respectively. In Figure 3.3.13 the values of d are depicted for those of the spectral exponent α used in Figure 3.3.11 and are compared with the theoretical value $d = 1/H$. The agreement is seen to be excellent from which we conclude that the random paths with inverse power-law spectra are self-affine fractal curves.

Panchev (1971) established a relation between the index of the structure function of a time series with an inverse power-law spectrum and the spectral exponent, which in the present case yields $\alpha = 2H + 1$. Thus the fractal dimension of a stochastic trajectory generated by a colored noise process with an inverse power-law spectrum is given by

$$d = 2/(\alpha - 1) \ . \qquad\qquad (3.3.26)$$

Since $0 < H < 1$ the inverse power law index is $1 < \alpha < 3$. For $\alpha > 3$ the Hausdorff dimension of the trajectory is equal to its topological dimension and the curve is no longer fractal. For $0 \le \alpha \le 1$ the scaling exponent is zero and d has an infinite value, i.e., the traditional expectation for stochastic processes is realized.

A number of other interesting conclusions can be reached regarding the statistical properties of the time series (3.3.19) with the spectrum (3.3.20) and for these the reader is referred to Osborne and Provenzale (1988).

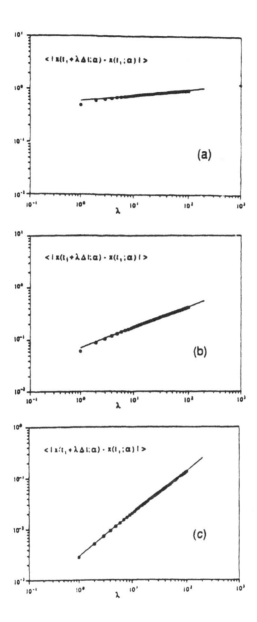

Figure 3.3.12.   The three straight lines correspond to $\alpha = 1.0$, 1.75 and 2.75 with the slope values from (3.3.25) given by $H \cong 0.1$, 0.39 and 0.84, respectively.

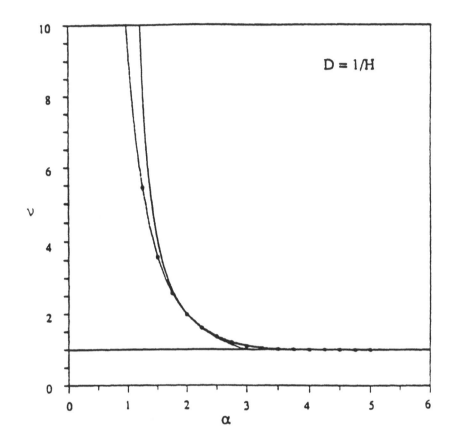

Figure 3.3.13. The fractal dimension d, determined as the inverse of the scaling exponent, versus the spectral exponent α. These results indicate the fractal and self-affine nature of the random noises studied here. The values of the fractal dimension $d = 1/H$ are in excellent agreement with the values of the correlation dimension shown in Figure 3.3.11. The solid and the dashed lines are theoretical relationships for respectively "perfect" and truncated power law spectra and are discussed in the text.

4. REVIEW OF SOME BIOMEDICAL APPLICATIONS OF THE RECONSTRUCTION TECHNIQUE

In Chapters 2 and 3 we have attempted to develop some rather difficult mathematical concepts and techniques in a way that would make their importance self-evident in a biomedical context. In the present section we take a single method, the reconstruction technique, and review how it has been applied to problems of biomedial interest and argue for its continued refinement and application in these areas. The list of examples is representative rather than exhaustive, but a rather extensive bibliography is attempted. This reconstruction technique is important because it provides a way to extract the greatest amount of modeling information from the data. The attractor that is reconstructed from the data is shown to clearly distinguish between uncorrelated noise and chaos, and since the ways to control systems contaminated by such noise are quite different from those manifesting fluctuations due to low-order nonlinear interactions, being able to distinguish between the two can be crucial. When such an attractor can be reconstructed from a time series it explicitly shows the number of variables required to faithfully model the phenomenon of interest.

In this chapter we span the realm of activity from that of the single neuron, through complex biochemical reactions to the social influence of epidemiology. In all these cases we see the rich dynamic structure of chaotic attractors and find that scientists have been able to exploit the concepts of nonlinear dynamics to answer some of the fundamental questions that were left unanswered or ambiguous using more traditional techniques. Let us examine epidemiology to begin our review of these activities.

Infectious diseases may be divided into those caused by microparasites such as viruses, bacteria and protozoa and those caused by macroparasites such as helminths and arthropods. Childhood epidemics of microparasitic infections such as mumps and chicken pox show almost periodic yearly outbreaks and those cyclic patterns of an infection have been emphasized in a number of studies (Anderson, Grenfelt and May, 1984) In Figure 4.0.1 is depicted the number of reported cases of infection each month for measles, chicken pox and mumps in New York City and measles in Baltimore. The obvious irregularities in these data have usually been explained in terms of stochastic models (Bartlett, 1960; Anderson, 1982), but the more recent applications of chaotic dynamics to these data have resulted in a number of interesting results. In Section 4.1 we review the analysis of Schaffer and Kott's (1985) analysis of the data in Figure 4.0.1.

A recent *research news* article in *Science* by R. Pool points out that the outbreaks of measles in New York City followed a curious pattern before the introduction of mass

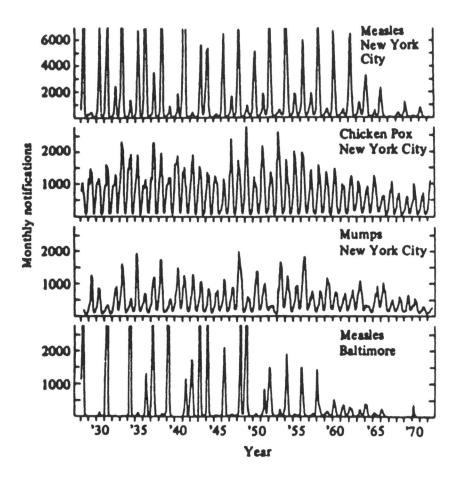

Figure 4.0.1. The monthly reported cases of measles, chicken pox and mumps in New York and measles in Baltimore in the periods 1928-72 (from London & Yorke, 1973).

vaccinations. When children returned to school each winter there was a sudden surge of infections corresponding to the periods the student remained indoors exchanging germs. Over and above this yearly cycle there occurred a bi-yearly explosion in the number of cases of measles with a factor of five to ten increase in the number of cases reported - sometimes as many as 10,000 cases a month.

He points out that this biennial cycle did not appear until after 1945. Prior to this, although the yearly peak occurred each winter, there did not seem to be any alternating pattern of mild and severe years. In the period 1928 to 1944 there was no organized pattern of mild and severe years; a relatively severe winter might be following by two mild ones, or vice versa. This is the irregularity that is arguably described by means of chaos.

It should be pointed out that these dramatic yearly fluctuations were ended with the implementation of a vaccination program in the early 1960's.

If we attempt to model physiological structures as complex systems arising out of the interaction of fundamental units, then it stands to reason that certain clinically observed failures in physiological regulation occur because of the failure of one or more of these fundamental units. One example of such a system is the mammalian central nervous system, and the question that immediately comes to mind is whether this system can display chaotic behavior? Rapp et al. (1985) present experimental evidence that strongly suggest that spontaneous chaotic behavior does occur. In the same vein Hayashi, Ishizuka, Ohta and Hirakawa (1982) show that sinusoidal electrical stimulation of the giant internodel cell of the freshwater algae *Nitella flexilis* causes entrainment, quasiperiodic behavior and chaos just as did the two oscillator model of the heart discussed in Chapter 3. We review both of these examples in Section 4.2.

The first dynamical system that was experimentally shown to manifest a rich variety of dynamics involved nonequilibrium, chemical reactions. Arneodo, Argoul, Richetti and Roux (1988) comment that one of the most common features of these chemical reactions is the alternating sequence of periodic and chaotic states, the Bebousov-Zhabotinskii reaction being the most throughly studied of the oscillating chemical reactions. We briefly indicate some of the experimental evidence for the existence of chaos in well-controlled nonequilibrium reactions in Section 4.3

There are a number of mathematical models of the heart (cf. Chapter 3), with an imaginative array of assumed physical and biological characteristics. In Section 4.4 we display some of the laboratory data that suggests that the electrical properties of the mammalian heart are manifestations of a chaotic attractor (Kobayashi and Musha, 1982;

182

Goldberger et al., 1985). One such indication comes from the time series interbeat intervals (RR), i.e., the number of R waves in the electrocardiographic signal. The ordered set of RR intervals form a suitable times series when the RR interval magnitude is plotted versus the interval number in the sequence of heart beats. We also indicate how to determine the fractal dimension of this time series.

4.1   The Dynamics of Epidemics

As pointed out by Schaffer and Kott (1985) discussions over the relative importance of deterministic and stochastic processes in regulating the incidence of disease have divided students of population dynamics. These authors show that much of the contention is more apparent than real, and is a consequence of how certain data are processed. Spectral analysis has been a traditional tool for discriminating between these two contributors to a given time series, e.g. those in Figure 4.0.1. We learned in Section 3.3, however, that even though some systems are completely deterministic their spectra may be very broad, i.e., indistinguishable from random noise (Crutchfield, Donnelly, Farmer, Jones, Packard and Shaw, 1980). We also saw that in other cases the spectrum can have a few sharp peaks superimposed on a broadband background. These peaks can be interpreted as phase coherence in the system dynamics (Farmer et al., 1980). Thus it is not possible by spectral means alone to distinguish deterministic (chaotic) dynamics from periodic motion contaminated by uncorrelated noise. We further saw that calculating a correlation dimension is also not sufficient to distinguish a chaotic from a correlated random time series. The correlation dimension indicates that the time series is fractal, but in itself it cannot determine the cause of the lack of a characteristic time scale. It could be correlations in a random process or it could be a chaotic attractor underlying the system dynamics. To distinguish between these options Schaffer and Kott applied the attractor reconstruction method discussed in the preceding chapter to epidemiological data sets.

There are a number of models that partition a population into a set of categories and describe the development of an epidemic by means of differential equations involving the interactions of the members of one category with those of another. The state variables are the number of individuals in each of the assigned categories: 1. *susceptibles (S)*; 2. *exposed (E)* (infected) 3. *infectious (I)* and 4. *recovered (R)* (immune)(London and Yorke, 1973; Dietz, 1976; Anderson and May, 1982). These four state variables give rise to the SEIR model for epidemics (Schaffer, 1989):

$$\dot{S}(t) = m[1 - S(t)] - bS(t)I(t) \ , \tag{4.1.1}$$

$$\dot{E}(t) = b\,S(t)I(t) - (m+a)E(t) \ , \tag{4.1.2}$$

$$\dot{I}(t) = aE(t) - (m+g)I(t) \ . \tag{4.1.3}$$

The fourth variable has been eliminated from this description by assuming that the total population is kept constant. Here, m^{-1} is the average life expectancy, a^{-1} is the average latency period, and g^{-1} is the average infectious period. The contact rate b is the average number of susceptibles contacted yearly per infective.

Most epidemiologists work with this model, or a variant of it whether they believe in chaos or not. Traditionally, they have examined simple regular solutions to these models. It is not difficult to choose parameter values to produce a two year low/high cycle that resembles the New York City history of measles from 1945 to 1963 as discussed by Pool. The regularity in these solutions do not faithfully represent the variability in the data, however, so that epidemiologists often introduce noise to randomize things. Schaffer and colleagues have demonstrated that the introduction of noise is not necessary to produce irregular infection patterns. For particular values of the parameters in the SEIR model they have produced computer simulations of measles epidemics closely resembling those seen in the New York City data. Before assigning values to the parameters m, a, g and b and solving the set (4.1.1) - (4.1.3), let us turn to the analysis of the data.

The number of cases of measles shown in Figure 4.0.1 are taken from London and York (1973) and are those reported monthly by physicians for the cities of New York and Baltimore for the years 1928 to 1963. Not all cases were reported because reporting was voluntary, so that Yorke and London estimate that the reported cases are between a factor five and seven below the actual number. In the spectra given in Figure 4.1.1 we see a number of peaks superimposed on a noisy background. The most prominent peak coincides with a yearly cycle with most cases occurring during the winter. The secondary peaks at 2 and 3 years are obtained by an appropriate smoothing of the data.

These data were also plotted using Taken's reconstruction technique as phase plots of $N(t)$, $N(t+\tau)$, $N(t+2\tau)$ when N is the number of cases per month and τ is a two to three month shift in the time axis. In Figure 4.1.2 and 4.1.3 we show the phase portraits obtained using the smoothed data. Schaffer and Kott point out that for both New York and Baltimore most of the trajectory traced out by the data lies on the surface of a cone with its vertex near the origin. They conclude by inspection of these figures that the attractor is an essentially two-dimensional object embedded in three dimensions.

184

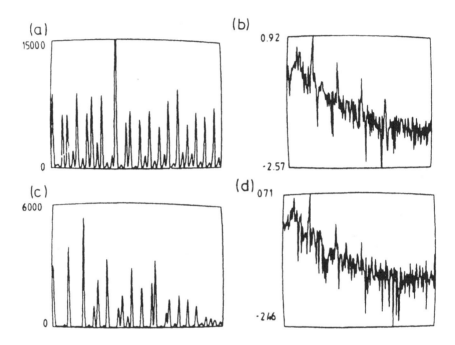

Figure 4.1.1. Epidemics of measles in New York and Baltimore. Left: The numbers of cases reported monthly by physicians from 1928 to 1963. Right: Power spectra (from Schaffer & Kott, 1985 with permission).

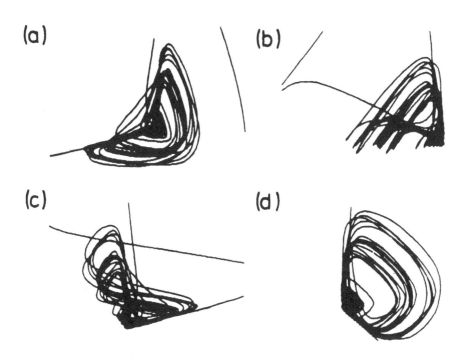

Figure 4.1.2. Reconstructed trajectory for the New York data (smoothed and interpolated). The motion suggests a unimodal 1-D map in the presence of noise. *a-d*. The data embedded in three dimensions and viewed from different perspectives (from Schaffer, 1985 with permission).

186

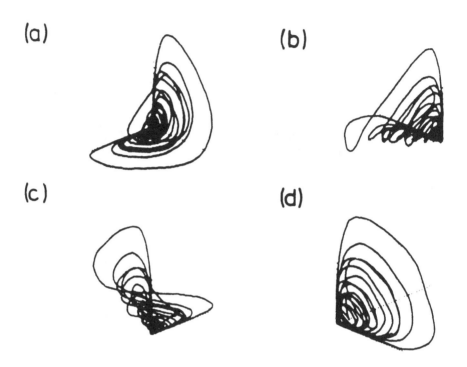

(a)

(b)

(c)

(d)

Figure 4.1.3. Reconstructed trajectory for the Baltimore data. The 1-D map is very steep and compressed. Order of photographs as in Figure 4.1.2 (from Schaffer, 1985 with permission).

This estimate is made more quantitative using the method of Grassberger and Procaccia (1983a, b) to calculate the correlation dimension. In Figure 4.1.4 we see that the dimension asymptotes to a value of approximately 2.5 as the embedding dimension is increased to five.

Let us now return to the SEIR model of epidemics. For measles in the large cities of rich countries, $m^{-1} \approx 10^2$, $a^{-1} \approx 10^{-1}$, and $g^{-1} \approx 10^{-2}$.[3] As given by (4.1.1) - (4.1.3) the solution to the SEIR model as determined by the value of the rate of infection Q:

$$Q = ba/[(m+a)(m+g)] \ .$$ (4.1.4)

If $Q < 1$ the disease dies out; if $Q > 1$, it persists at a constant level and is said to be endemic. At long times neither of these solutions captures the properties of the attractors shown in Figures 4.1.2 and 4.1.3, i.e., the observation of recurrent epidemics is at variance with the predictions of the SEIR model as formulated above.

To study the effect of seasonality Schaffer (1985) replaces the contact rate b in (4.1.1) and (4.1.2) with a periodic function

$$b(t) = b_1[1 + \cos 2\pi t] \ .$$ (4.1.5)

For this form of the contact rate the solution to the SEIR-model has period-doubling bifurcations leading to chaos (Aron and Schwartz, 1984; Schwartz and Smith, 1983; 1988). If we now proceed as with the data and take the solution for the number of exposed or infectives and apply the reconstruction technique Schaffer obtains the results shown in the top row of Figure 4.1.5. In this figure the attractors generated by the data are compared with that produced by the SEIR model. The resemblance among the attractors is obvious. The second row depicts the attractors as seen from above. From this perspective the essential two-dimensional nature of the flow field is most evident. Poincaré sections are taken by plotting the intersection of the attractor with a transverse line drawn through each of the three attractors. It is seen that these sections are V-shaped half lines, demonstrating that the flow is confined to a nearly two-dimensional conical surface. A one-dimensional map was constructed by plotting the sequential intersecting points against one another yielding the nearly single humped maps shown in the final row Figure 4.1.5. These maps for the New York and Baltimore measle data depict a strong correlation between consecutive intersections. When a similar analysis was made of the chicken pox and mumps data no such correlation was observed, i.e., the plot yielded a random spray of points.

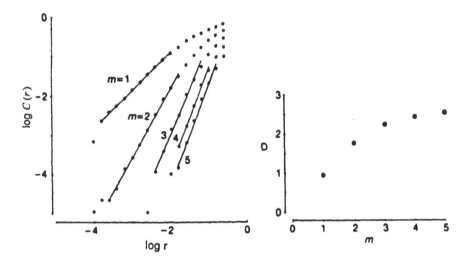

Figure 4.1.4. Estimating the fractal dimension for measles epidemics in New York. Left: The correlation integral $C(r)$ plotted against the length scale r for different embeddings m of the data. Right: Slope of the log-log plot against embedding dimension (from Schaffer, 1985 with permission).

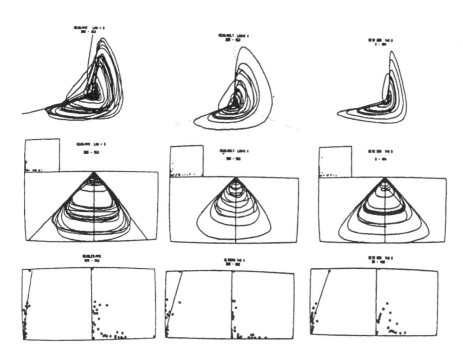

Figure 4.1.5. Measles epidemics real and imagined. Top row. Orbits reconstructed form the numbers of infective individuals reported monthly with three-point smoothing and interpolation with cubic splines (Schaffer and Kott, 1985). Time lag for reconstructions indicated in photos. Middle row. Orbits viewed from above (main part of the figures) and sliced with a plane (vertical line) normal to the paper. Poincaré sections shown in the small boxes at upper left. Bottom row. One of the Poincaré sections magnified (left) and resulting 1-D map (right). In each case, 36 years of data are shown. Left column: data from New York City. Middle column: data from Baltimore. Right column: SEIR equations with parameters as in Figure 4.1.2 save $b_1 = 0.28$ (from Schaffer, 1985 with permission).

The failure of the chicken pox and mumps data to yield a low dimensional attractor in phase space lead Schaffer and Kott to investigate the effects of uncorrelated noise on a known deterministic map. The measure they used to determine the nature of the attractor was the one-dimensional map from the Poincaré surface of section. They argued that the random distribution of points observed in the data could well be the result of a map of the form

$$X_{n+1} = (1 + Z_n)F(X_n) \qquad\qquad (4.1.6)$$

where $F(X_n)$ is the mapping function and Z_n is a discrete random variable with Gaussian statistics of prescribed mean and variance. They showed that the multiplicative noise Z_n could totally obscure the underlying map $F(X_n)$ when the dynamics are periodic. However as the system bifurcates and moves towards chaos the effect of the noise is reduced, becoming negligible when chaos is reached. Thus they conclude, "that whereas noise can easily obscure the underlying determinism for systems with simple dynamics, this turns out not to be the case if the dynamics are complex." This result is at variance with the earlier interpretation of Bartlett (1960) that the observed spectrum for measles resulted from the interaction between a stochastic environment and weakly damped deterministic oscillations. Olsen and Degn (1985) support the conclusions of Schaffer and Kott, stating:

"The conclusion that measles epidemics in large cities may be chaotic due to a well defined, albeit unknown mechanism is also supported by the analysis of measles data from Copenhagen yielding a one-dimensional humped map almost identical to the ones found from the New York and Baltimore data."

Hence we have seen that the reconstruction method is not only useful when the data yield a low-dimensional attractor, but also when it does not. That is to say that certain of the ideas in nonlinear dynamics conjoined with the older concepts of stochastic equations, can explain why certain data sets do *not* yield one-dimensional maps. These insights will become sharper through additional examples.

In order not to leave the reader with the impression that this interpretation of the data is uniformly accepted by the epidemiological community we mention the criticism of Aron (1989) and Schwartz (1985). Much of the debate centers on the contact rate parameter, which because it varies through the year, must be estimated indirectly. Aron contends that the models are extremely sensitive to parameters such as the contact rate, and the variation in these parameters over 30 to 40 years could produce the fluctuations [see Pool (1989)]. Schwartz argues with Aron and cautions against the over-use of such simplified models as the SEIR, since it does not yield *quantitative* agreement with the real world situation. Pool's article gives a clear exposition of the present state of the debate.

4.2   Chaotic Neurons

The accepted theory of the generation and propagation of the excitation of nerve and muscle cells involves electrochemical processes localized in the membranes of those cells. The movement of the nerve pulse corresponds to the movement of small ions. Nerve excitation is transmitted throughout the nerve fiber which itself is part of the *nerve cell* who is known as a *neuron*. The neuron is in most respects quite similar to other cells in that it contains a nucleus and cytoplasm. It is distinctive in that long, threadlike tendrils emerge from the cell body, and those numerous projections branch out into still finer extensions. These are the *dendrites* that form a branching tree of ever more slender threads not unlike the fractal trees discussed earlier. One such thread does not branch and often extends for several meters even though it is still part of a single cell. This is the *axon* which is the nerve fiber in the typical nerve. [See e.g. Valkenshtein, 1983 or Asinov, 1963.] Excitations (depolarization waves) in the dendrites essentially always travel toward the cell body in a living system whereas in the axon they always travel away from the cell body.

In 1852 the German physician-physicist Helmholtz first measured the speed of the nerve impulse by stimulating a nerve at different points and recording the time it took for the muscle to which it was connected to respond . It was not until half a century later that Bernstein worked out the membrane theory of excitation.

It has been known for some time that the activity of a nerve is always accompanied by electrical phenomena. Whether it is external excitation of a nerve or the transmission of a message from the brain, electrical impulses are observed in the corresponding axon. As pointed out by Kandel (1979), because of the difficulty in examining patterns of interconnections in the human brain, there has been a major effort on the part of neurologists to develop animal models for studying how interacting systems of neurons give rise to behavior . There appears, for example, to be no fundamental differences in structure, chemistry or function between the neurons and their interconnections in man and those of a squid, a snail or a leech. However neurons do vary in size, position, shape, pigmentation, firing patterns and the chemical substances by which they transmit information to other cells. Here we are most interested in the differences in the firing patterns taken for example from the abdominal ganglion of *aphysia*. As Kandel (1979) points out certain cells are normally "silent" where others are spontaneously active. As shown in Figure 4.2.1 some of the active ones fire regular action potentials, or nerve impulses, and others fire in recurrent brief bursts or pulse trains. These different patterns result from differences in the types of ionic currents generated by the membrane of the cell body of the neurons.

The rich dynamic structure of the neuron firing patterns has lead to their being modeled by nonlinear dynamical systems. In Figure 4.2.1 the normally silent neuron can be viewed as a fixed point of a dynamic system. The periodic pulse train is suggestive of a limit cycle and finally, the erratic bursting of random wave trains is not unlike the time series generated by certain chaotic attractors. This spontaneous behavior of the individual neurons may be modified by driving the neurons with external excitations. This will be done subsequently. It is also possible that the normal activity can be modified through changes in internal control parameters of the isolated system.

Rapp et al. (1985) speculate that transitions among fixed point, periodic and chaotic attractors by varying system control parameters may be observed clinically in failures of physiological regulation. The direction of the transition is still the source of some controversy, as mentioned before with regard to the heart, it remains unresolved whether certain pathologies are a transition from normally ordered periodic behavior to abnormal chaos, or from normally chaotic behavior to abnormal periodicity. In the earlier cardiac context the author supports the latter position (Goldberger and West, 1987; West and Goldberger, 1987a,b) There also seems to be evidence accumulating in a number of other contexts, the present one included, to support the view that the observed rich dynamic structure in normal behavior is a consequence of chaotic attractors, and the apparent rhythmic dynamics are the phase coherence in the attractors. Rapp et al. (1985) present experimental evidence that spontaneous chaotic behavior does in fact occur in neurons.

In their study Rapp et al. (1985) recorded the time between action potentials (interspike intervals), of spontaneously active neurons in the precentral and postcentral gyri (the areas immediately anterior and posterior to the central fissure) of the squirrel monkey brain. The set of measured interspike intervals $\{t_j\}$, $j = 1, 2, ..., M$, was used to define a set of vectors $\mathbf{X}_j = (t_j, t_{j+1}, \cdots, t_{j+m-1})$ in an m-dimensional embedding space. These vectors are used to calculate the correlational integral of Grassberger and Procaccia (1983a,b) discussed in Chapter 3.

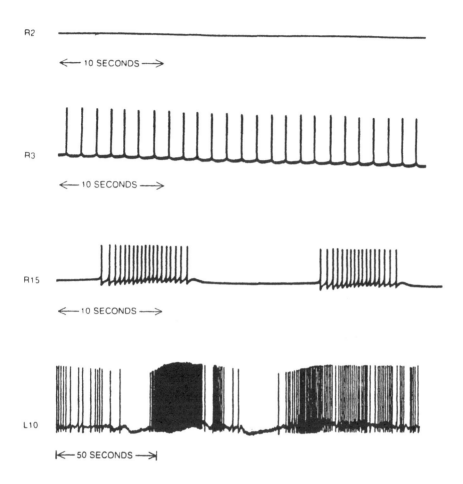

Figure 4.2.1. Firing patterns of identified neurons in *Aplysia's* abdominal ganglion are portrayed. R2 is normally silent, R3 has a regular beating rhythm, R15 a regular bursting rhythm and L10 an irregular bursting rhythm. L10 is a command cell that controls other cells in the sytem.

To determine the correlational dimension from the interspike interval data one must determine a scaling region in $C_m(r)$ between the noise at small r and the constant value of unity for larger r. The plateau in the slope versus $ln\, C_m(r)$ graphs in Figure 4.2.2 defines the scaling region. In Figure 4.2.2b we observe a plateau region for $ln\, C_m(r)$ in the interval $(-4.5, -2.5)$ for $m = 15$ to $m = 20$. In Figure 4.2.2d we see that no such plateau region is reached up to an embedding dimension of $m = 40$ indicating that this time series cannot be distinguished from uncorrelated random noise. Of ten neurons measured, three were clearly described by low dimensional fractal time series, two were ambiguous, and five could be modeled by uncorrelated random noise.

Rapp et al., (1985) drew the following two conclusions from this study:

"1. . . . the spontaneous activity of some simian cortical neurons, at least on occasion, may be chaotic; 2. . . .irrespective of any question of chaos, the dimension of the attractor governing the behavior can, at least for some neurons for some of the time, be very low."

For these last neurons we have the remarkable result that as few as three or four variables may be sufficient to model the neuronal dynamics if in fact the source of their fractal nature is a low-dimensional attractor. It would have been reckless to anticipate this result, but we now see that in spite of the profound complexity of the mammalian central nervous system the dynamics of some of its components may be describable by low-dimensional dynamic systems. Thus even though we do not know what the dynamic relations for these neurons systems might be, the fact that they do manifest such relatively simple dynamical behavior, bodes well for the eventual discovery of the underlying dynamics laws.

The next level of dynamic complexity still involving only a single neuron is its response when subjected to stimulation. This is a technique that was mature long before nonlinear dynamics was a defined concept in biology. We review some of the studies here because it is clear that many neurons capable of self-sustained oscillations are sinusoidally driven as part of the hierarchal structure in the central nervous system. The dynamics of the isolated neuron, whether periodic or chaotic, may well be modified through periodic stimulation. This has been found to be the case.

Hayashi, Nakao and Hirakawa (1982) were the first investigators to experimentally show evidence of chaotic behavior in a self-sustained oscillations of an excitable biological membrane under sinusoidal stimulation. The experiments were carried out on the giant internodal cell of the fresh water algae *Nitella flexilis*. A sinusoidal stimulation,

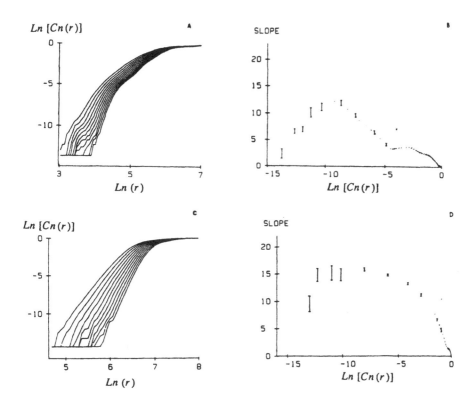

Figure 4.2.2. Estimation of attractor dimension. (a) Plot of $\log C_m(r)$ versus $\log r$, $m = 10$ to $m = 20$, for neuron A. (b) The corresponding plot of $d \log C_m(r)/d \log r$ as a function of $\log C_m(r)$, $m = 15$ to $m = 20$, for neuron A. The plateau exists between -4.5 and 2.5. The dimension of the attractor is estimated to be 3.5. (c) Plot of $\log C_m(r)$ versus $\log \varepsilon$ for neuron C, $m = 20$ to $m = 40$ in steps of two. (d) The plot of $d \log C_m(r)/d \log(r)$ as a function of $\log C_m(r)$ for neuron C, $m = 30$ to $m = 40$ in steps of two. No plateau is found up to embedding dimension $m = 40$ (from Rapp, Zimmerman, Albano, de Guzman and Greenbaum, 1985 with permission).

$A\cos\omega_i t + B$, was applied to the internodal cell which was firing repetitively. The DC outward current B was applied in order to stably maintain the repetitive firing which was sustained for 40 minutes. In Figure 4.2.3 the repetitive firing under the sinusoidal current stimulation is shown. In Figure 4.2.3a the firing current is seen to be one-to-one phase locked to the stimulating current. The phase plot of segmented peaks is shown in Figure 4.2.4a, where the stroboscopic mapping function is observed to converge on a point lying along a line of unit slope. In Figure 4.2.3b we see that the firing of the neuron has become aperiodic losing its entrainment to the stimulation. This in itself is not sufficient to establish the existence of a low-dimensional chaotic attractor. Additional evidence is required. The authors obtain this evidence by constructing the mapping function between successive maxima of the pulse train. For an uncorrelated random time series this mapping function is just a random spray of points, whereas for a chaotic time series this function is well defined. The mapping of sequential peaks depicted in Figure 4.2.4b reveals a single-valued mapping function. The slope of this function is less than −1 at its intersection with the line of unit slope. The lines in Figure 4.2.4b clearly indicate that the mapping function admits of a period three solution. Hayashi et al. (1982) then invoked a theorem due to Li and Yorke (1975) that states: ''period three implies chaos.'' They subsequently show that entrained, harmonic, quasiperiodic and chaotic responses of the self-sustained firing of the *Nitella* internodal cell occur for different values of the amplitude and frequency of the periodic external force (Hayashi, Nakao and Hirakawa, 1983). These same four categories of responses were obtained by Matsumoto, Aihara, Ichikawa and Tasaki (1984) using a squid giant axon.

The above group (Hayashi, Ishizuka, Ohta and Hirakawa, 1982) also investigated the periodic firing of the *Onchidium* giant neuron under sinusoidal stimulation (the pacemaker neuron from the marine pulmonate mollusk *Onchidium verraculatum*). The oscillatory response does not synchronize with the sinusoidal stimulation, but is instead aperiodic. The trajectory of the oscillation is shown in Figure 4.2.5 and we see that it is not a single closed curve but a filled region of phase space. This region is bounded by the trajectory of the larger action potentials. Here again the stroboscopic mapping function is useful for characterizing the type of chaos that is evident in Figure 4.2.5. The single-humped mapping function is shown in Figure 4.2.6 and is clearly quite similar to the one observed in Figure 4.2.4b for a different neuron. Again the maps allows for period three orbits and therefore chaos (Hayashi et al., 1983). Further studies by this group indicate that due to the form of the one-dimensional map the transition to chaos

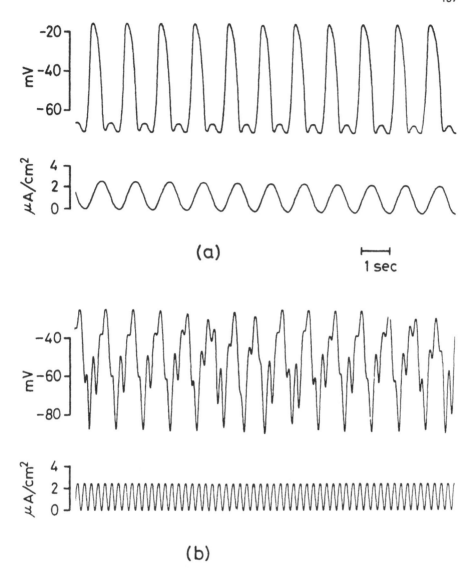

Figure 4.2.3. Entrainment and chaos in the sinusoidally stimulated internodal cell of
Nitella. (a) Repetitive firing (upper curve) synchronized with the periodic
current stimulation (lower curve). (b) Non-periodic response to periodic
stimulation (from Hayashi, Nakao and Hirakawa, 1982 with permission).

198

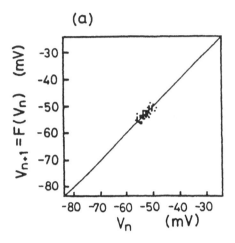

(a)

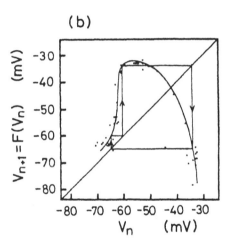

(b)

Figure 4.2.4. (a) and (b) are the stroboscopic transfer function obtained from Figure 4.2.3 (a) and (b) respectively. The membrane potential at each peak of the periodic stimulation was plotted against the preceding one. Period three is indicated graphically by arrows in (b) (from Hayashi, Nakao & Hirakawa, 1983 with permission).

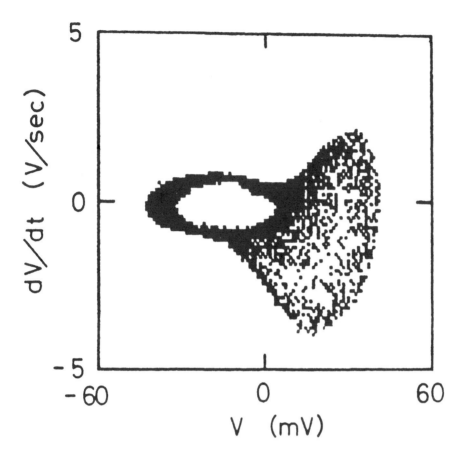

Figure 4.2.5. The trajectory of the nonperiodic oscillation. The trajectory is filling up a
finite region of the phase space. The oscillation of the membrane potential was differentiated by the differentiated circuit whose phase did not
shift in the frequency region below 40 Hz (from Hayashi et al., 1982 with
permission).

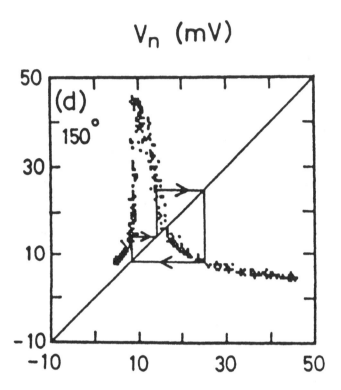

Figure 4.2.6. Stroboscopic transfer function of the chaotic response to periodic current stimulation in the Onchidium giant neuron. The plot was obtained in the same way as that of Figure 4.2.4c and 4.2.4d. The arrows indicate period three (from Hayashi et al., 1983 with permission).

occurs through intermittency.

Now that we have such compelling experimental evidence that the basic unit of the central nervous system has such a repertoire of dynamic responses it is reasonable to ask if the solutions to any models have these features. In the case of epidemics we observed that the SEIR model did capture the essential features found in the data. It has similarly been determined by Aihara, Matsumoto and Ikegaza (1984) that the numerical solutions to the periodically forced Hodgkin-Huxley equations also give rise to this array of dynamic responses. The Hodgkin-Huxley equations for the membrane potential difference V is

$$\frac{dV}{dt} = \left[I - \bar{g}_{Na} m^3 h (V - V_{Na}) - \bar{g}_K n^4 (V - V_K) - \bar{g}_L (V - V_L) \right] / C \qquad (4.2.1)$$

where the $\bar{g}_j$'s are the maximal ionic conductances and the V_j's are the reversal potentials for j = sodium (Na), potassium (N) and leakage current component (L); I is the membrane current density (positive outward); C is the membrane capacitance; m is the dimensionless sodium activation; h is the dimensionless sodium inactivation and n is the dimensionless potassium activation. The functions m, h and n satisfy their own rate equations that depend on V and the temperature, but we will not write these down here; see e.g. Aihara et al. (1984).

There was good agreement found between the time series of the experimental oscillations in the membrane potential of the periodically forced squid axon by Matsumoto et al. (1984) and those obtained in the numerical study by Aihara et al. (1984). The latter authors determined that there were two routes to chaos followed by the Hodgkin-Huxley equations: successive period doubling bifurcations and the formation of the intermittently chaotic oscillation from subharmonic synchronization. The former route had previously been analyzed by Rinzel and Miller (1980) for the autonomous Hodgkin-Huxley equations, whereas the present discussion focusses on the non-autonomous system. Aihara et al. (1984) reach the conclusion:

"Therefore, it is expected that periodic currents of various forms can produce the chaotic responses in the forced Hodgkin-Huxley oscillator and giant axon. This implies that neural systems of nonlinear neural oscillators connected by chemical and electrical synapses to each other can show chaotic oscillations and supply macroscopic fluctuations to the biological brain."

4.3   Chemical Chaos

Chemistry forms the basis of all biomedical phenomena. Hess and Markus (1987) point out that in biochemistry, oscillating dynamics play a prominent role in biological clock functions, in inter- and intracellular signal transmission, and in cellular differentiation. We should observe that certain solutions to the periodically forced Hodgkin-Huxley equation, that describe the chemically driven membrane potential in neurons, are chaotic. In chemical reactions there are certain species called reactants that are continuously converted to other species called products. In complex reactions there are often other species around, called intermediaries, whose concentration both increase and decrease during the course of the primary reaction. In simple reacting systems subject to diffusion the reactants, products and intermediaries normally approach a spatially uniform state, i.e., a state in which each species concentration approaches a different constant value in the reacting mixture. In the type of reaction considered by Rössler (1980) it was assumed that the chemical mixture is well stirred at all times so the reaction is independent of where in the mixture it occurs. That is to say that the effects of spatial diffusion are removed from the total rate of change of the reactant concentration and oscillations become possible. Such oscillating reactions have been widely studied in the past decade; see e.g. Hess (1977), Rapp (1979) and Olsen and Degn (1977).

In the Belousov-Zhabotinskii (BZ) reaction, mentioned earlier, the bifurcation behavior we have been discussing is clearly observed. In Figure 4.3.1 we see the transition from a steady state, of the "constant" concentration of bromide ions and ceruim ions, that persists for over 600 seconds, to a periodic state. A readable discussion of this reaction for the nonspecialist is given by Field (1987), wherein he points out that the control parameter (bifurcation parameter μ) is the amount of $BrCH(COOH)_2$ in the reacting vessel. One would have expected that the amplitude of the oscillating concentration would have started out small and gradually increased. Bifurcation theory offers an explanation as to why the oscillations appear at its full level rather than gradually increasing. The steady state remains locally stable until the control parameters exceeds a critical value at which point the steady state becomes unstable and makes a transition to a periodic state. This sudden change in behavior is characteristic of bifurcations in systems governed by nonlinear kinetics laws and evolving biological systems (Field, 1987; Taylor, 1983).

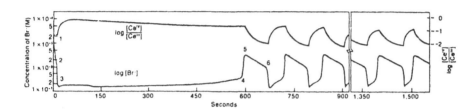

Figure 4.3.1. The Belousov-Zhabotinskii (BZ) reaction is the most fully understood chemical reaction that exhibits chemical organization. The general behavior of this reaction as the concentrations of bromide and cerium ions oscillate (from Field, 1987 with permission).

Simoyi et al. (1982) conducted experiments on the BZ reaction in a well-stirred reactor as a function of the flow rate of the chemicals through the reactor. In Figure 4.3.2 is depicted the observed bromide-ion potential time series for different values of the flow rate (the flow rate is the bifurcation parameter in this experiment). They, as well as Roux, Turner, McCormick and Swinney (1982), used the embedding theorems (Whitney, 1936; Takens, 1981) to justify reconstruction of the dynamic attractor from the single bromide-ion concentration (Field, 1987).

Thus, for sufficiently high values of the control parameter (flow rate) the attractor becomes chaotic. In Figure 4.3.3a is depicted a two-dimensional projection of the three-dimensional phase portrait of the attractor with the third axis normal to the plane of the page. A Poincaré surface of section is constructed by recording the intersection of the attractor with the dashed line to obtain the set of data points $\{X_n\}$. The mapping function shown in Figure (4.3.3b) is obtained using these data points. The one-humped form of the one-dimensional map clearly indicates the chaotic character of the attractor. These observations were thought to provide the first example of a physical system with many degrees of freedom that can be modeled in detail by a one-dimensional map. However, Olsen and Degn (1977) had observed chaos in the oscillating enzyme reaction: peroxidase-oxidase reaction in an open system some five years earlier. The next amplitude plot for this latter reaction does *not* yield the simple one-humped mapping function shown in Figure 4.3.3b, but rather has a "Cantor set-like" structure as shown in Figure 4.3.4. Olsen and Degn (1977) constructed a mathematical model containing the minimal chemical expressions for quadratic branchings. The results yielded periodic and chaotic oscillations closely resembling the experimental results. In Figure 4.3.4 the next amplitude plot of the chaotic solutions for the data is overlayed on the numerical solutions. As pointed out by Olsen (1983), "The dynamic behavior of the peroxidase-oxidase reaction may thus be more complex than the behavior previously reported for the BZ reaction" (Simoyi et al., 1982; Roux et al., 1982; Takens, 1981).

Yet a third chemical reaction manifesting a rich dynamic behavior is glycolysis under periodic excitation. Markus, Kuschwitz and Hess (1985) examined the properties of periodic and aperiodic glycolytic oscillations in yeast extracts under sinusoidal glucose input. They used a variety of methods to analyze these reactions including spectral analysis, phase space reconstruction, Poincaré surface of section and the determination of the Lyapunov exponent for the attractor dynamics. They used a two-enzyme glycolytic

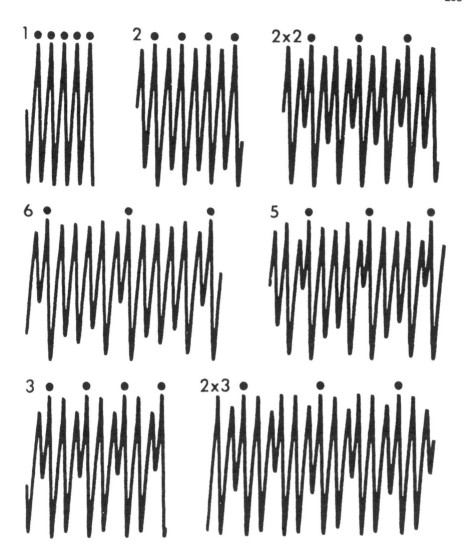

Figure 4.3.2. Observed bromide-ion potential series with periods τ (115 s), 2τ, $2\times2\tau$, 6τ, 5τ, 3τ, and $2\times3\tau$; the dots above the time series are separated by one period (from Simoyi et al., 1982 with permission).

206

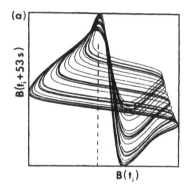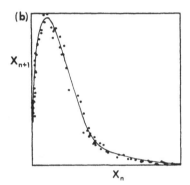

Figure 4.3.3. (a) A two-dimensional projection of a three-dimensional phase portrait for the chaotic state reconstructed from the Belousov-Zhabotinskii chemical reaction. (b) A one dimensional map constructed from the data in (a) (from Simoyi et al., 1982 with permission).

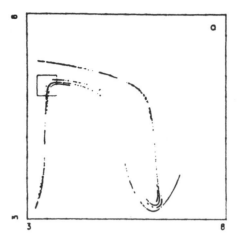

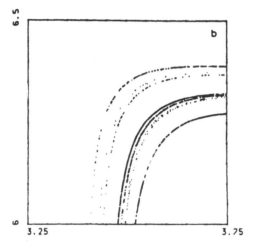

Figure 4.3.4. Next amplitude plot of the oscillators observed in the peroxidase-oxidase reaction. (a) 3000 maxima have been computed. The first of these maxima is preceded by 100 maxima that were discarded. (b) Magnification of the square region shown in (a) (from Olsen, 1983 with permission).

model to predict a rich variety of periodic responses and strange attractors from numerical solutions of the equations and then experimentally confirmed the existence of these predicted states.

The experiments were conducted with cell-free extracts of commercial bakers' yeast (Saccharomyces cerevisiae) (ph 6.4, 22-23°, 20-27 mg protein/ml) by continuous and periodic injection of 0.3 M glucose and recording the NADH fluorescence (F). In Figure 4.3.5 their experimental results are depicted. The lower curve indicates the periodic input flux, and the upper curve shows a typical train of response variations with no discernible period. Using the upper curve as our data set the power spectra density indicates a broad brand spectrum indicative of noise (randomness) on which a number of sharp peaks are superimposed indicating order. As we now know the presence of these two features are indicative of chaos in the time series. If T_e is the period of the input flux then F_n defined as the value of $F(t)$ at time $t = nT_e$ can be used to obtain the "stroboscopic transfer" function. The nonlinear map such as shown in Figure 4.3.3 and 4.3.4. In Figure 4.3.6 two determinations of the one-dimensional map are depicted. In plot (a) an oscillation with a response period equal to $3T_e$ is shown, wherein the map consists of three distinct patches of data points. In plot (b) we see from the single humped map that the time series is aperiodic. Markus et al. point out that this transfer function allows the determination of a sequence of points having the same periodicity as plot (a), namely those indicated by 1, 2 and 3. According to the Li-York theorem (1975), this transfer function thus admits of chaos. Further verification of the chaotic nature of the time series was made through the evaluation of the Lyapunov characteristic exponent λ. As we mentioned in the Introduction the Lyapunov exponent is interpreted as the average rate of growth of information as the system evolves. A chaotic system is one possessing a positive Lyapunov exponent and thereby has a positive rate of increase of macroscopic information. They obtain $\lambda \approx 0.95$ bits as the rate of growth of information during chaotic response.

4.4 Cardiac Chaos

As we discussed in Section 3.1 there are several areas of the mammalian heart capable of spontaneous, rhythmic self-excitation, but under physiologic conditions the normal pacemaker is the sino-atrial (SA) node. The SA mode is a small mass of pacemaker cells embedded in the right atrial wall near the entrance of the superior vena

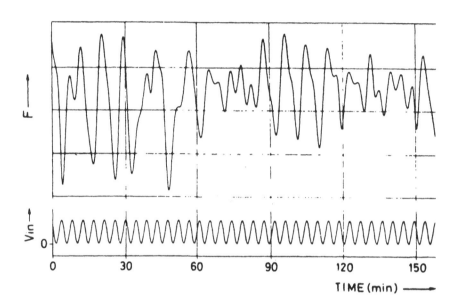

Figure 4.3.5. Measured NADH fluorescence (upper curve) of yeast extract under sinusoidal glucose input flux (lower curve) (from Markus et al., 1985 with permission).

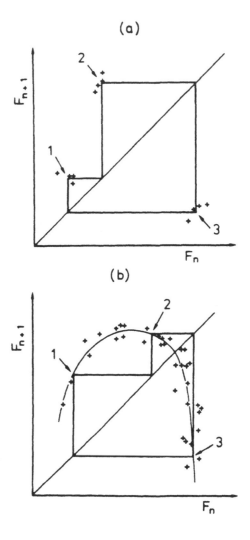

Figure 4.3.6. Stroboscopic transfer function for a periodic response at $\omega_e = 3.02\,\omega_0$ (a) and for chaos at $\omega_e = 2.76\,\omega_0$ (b). The plus signs (+) indicate the signal F_{n+1} (arbitrary units) measured at time $(n+1)\,T_c$ versus the signal F_n at time nT_e, where T_e is the input flux period. The solid curve in panel (b) is an interpolated transfer function. The period in panel (a) is $3T_e$ and the transfer function in panel (b) admits the same period. These periodicities are indicated in both panels by vertical and horizontal lines and by the numbers (from Markus et al. 1985 with permission).

cava. An impulse generated by the SA node spreads through the atrial muscle (triggering atrial contraction). The depolarization wave then spreads through the atrioventricular (AV) node and down the His-Purkinjé system into the right and left ventricles. There are a large number of both linear and nonlinear mathematical models describing this process of conduction between the SA and AV nodes. Here we show how a number of experimental studies have used the new nonlinear tools to distinguish between chaos and noise (Keener, 1987; West et al., 1985; Guevara and Glass, 1982; Ritzenberg, Adam and Cohen, 1984; Ikeda, 1982), and to help understand the physiological dynamics.

The experimental technique of externally stimulating a neuron to induce behavior that enables the experimenter to deduce its intrinsic dynamics has also been applied by Glass et al. (1983) to aggregates of spontaneously beating cultured cardiac cells. These aggregates of embryonic cells of chick heart were exposed to brief single and periodic current pulses and the response recorded. A fundamental assumption of this work is that changes in the cardiac rhythm can be associated with bifurcations in the qualitative dynamics of the type of mathematical models we have been considering. The analysis of Glass et al. (1983) makes the three explicit assumptions:

"(i) A cardiac oscillator under normal conditions can be described by a system of ordinary differential equations with a single unstable steady state and displaying an asymptotically stable limit cycle oscillation which is globally attracting except for a set of singular points of measure zero."

"(ii) Following a short perturbation, the time course of the return to the limit cycle is much shorter than the spontaneous period of oscillation or the time between periodic pulses."

"(iii) The topological characteristics of the phase transition curve (PTC) change in stereotyped ways as the stimulus strength increases."

Denote the phase of the oscillator immediately before the ith stimulus of a periodic stimulation with a period τ by ϕ_i. The recursion relation is

$$\phi_{i+1} = g(\phi_i) + \tau/T_0 , \qquad (4.4.1)$$

where $g(\phi)$ is the experimentally determined phase response function for that stimulus strength and $g(\phi+j) = g(\phi)+j$ for an integer j and T_0 is the period of the limit cycle. Equation (4.4.1) measures the contraction of the aggregate as a function of the phase of the contraction at the time of the perturbation. Using the phase resetting data a Poincaré map was constructed to determine the phase transition function (cf. Figure 4.4.1). This

212

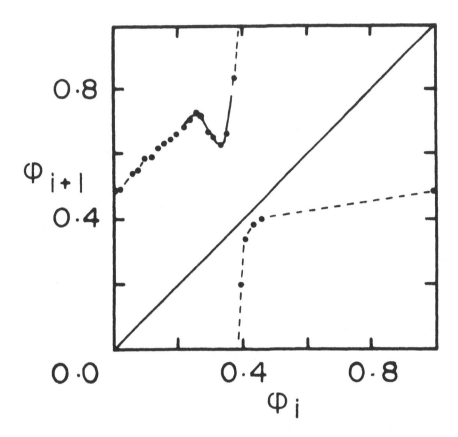

Figure 4.4.1. The new phase of the cardiac oscillator following a stimulation is plotted against the old phase, the resulting curve is called the phase transition curve. This is denoted by $g(\phi)$ in the text (from Glass et al., 1983 with permission).

is done by plotting the new phase following a stimulation against the old phase, the resulting curve is called the phase transition curve. The theoretical equation (4.4.1) is now iterated, using the experimentally determined $g(\phi)$, to compute the response of the aggregate to periodic stimulation. The observed responses to such perturbation are phase locking, period doubling and chaotic dynamics as the frequency of the periodic driver is increased.

The above authors do *not* attribute the observed irregularity to deterministic chaotic dynamics alone, but also argue that the observed effects can be strongly influenced by biological and environmental noise. Also that prolonged periodic stimulation of the aggregate changes the response properties of the aggregate.

In summary, the dynamics in response to periodic stimulation are predicted by iterating the experimentally derived map and bears a close resemblance to that observed experimentally. Glass et al. (1983) point out that the experimentally observed dynamics show patters similar to many commonly observed cardiac arrhythmias. Ikeda, Tsuruta and Sato (1981) use the properties of the phase response model to explain ventricular parasystoles. Guevara and Glass (1982) associate intermittent or variable AV block with the complex irregular behavior characteristic of chaotic dynamics observed in the phase response model.

The above authors (Glass et al., 1983) unanimously associate the chaotic dynamics with pathological rather than normal cardiac behavior. The same conclusions were reached by Ritzenberg, Adam and Cohen (1984) using the electrocardiogram and arterial blood pressure traces of noradrenaline-treated-dogs. Noradrenaline was found to produce variations in these traces that repeat themselves with regular periods of integral numbers of heart beats, an effect reminiscent of subharmonic bifurcation. A next amplitude plot of the T-waves is depicted in Figure 4.4.2. If this plot is viewed as a one-dimensional map then it is monotonic and hence invertible and therefore in itself does not provide evidence for the occurrence of chaos. Oono, Kohda and Yamazaki (1980) analyze the pulses of a patient suffering from arrhythmia and also construct a next amplitude plot of T-waves. The map in Figure 4.4.3 clearly shows that the arrhythmia of this patient is characterized by an orbit of period three. This suggests that Figure 4.4.2 may be more consistently interpreted as two distinct blobs rather than as a continuous map.

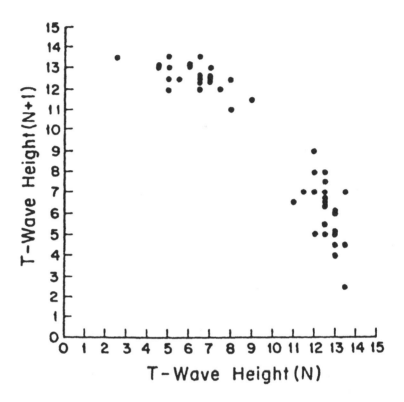

Figure 4.4.2. The height to the $N+1^{st}$ T-wave is plotted against the height of the Nth T-wave during 48 beats of an episode of period doubling (from Oono, Kohda and Yamazaki, 1980 with permission).

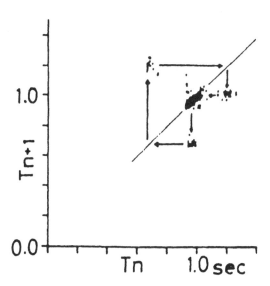

Figure 4.4.3. A next amplitude plot of T-wave maximum yields a period three orbit from a patient with an arrhythmia (from Oono et al., 1980 with permission).

Let us again consider the electrical activity of the normal heart, where the potential difference between various points on the surface of the body is called the electrocardiogram (ECG). The ECG time series consists of the P-wave, the QRS complex and the T-wave (cf. Figure 4.4.4). The first component reflects the excitation of the atria, the second that of the ventricles (His-Purkinjé network) and the third is associated with recovery of the initial electrical state of the ventricles (see Section 2.4). Traditional wisdom and everyday experience tells us that the ECG time series is periodic; however, quantitative analysis of the time series reveals a number of irregularities in the ECG record.

In Section 3.1 we presented a set of coupled nonlinear differential equations to model certain features of the cardiac dynamics. This model, based on a generalization of the cardiac oscillator (West et al., 1984) of van der Pol and van der Mark (1928,1929), gives a qualitative fit to the ECG time series, but does not account for the observed fluctuations in the data. The question arises as to whether these fluctuations are the result of the oscillations being unpredictably perturbed by the cardiac environment, or are a consequence of cardiac dynamics being given by a chaotic attractor, or both. As we mentioned there are several techniques available from dynamical systems theory that enable us to distinguish between these two possibilities. Spectral analysis, temporal autocorrelation function and the phase space reconstruction method are qualitative whereas the correlation dimension, Lyapunov exponents and Kolmogorov entropy are quantitative.

In Section 2.4 we discussed the power spectrum of the QRS complex of a normal heart and discussed the hypothesis that the fractal structure of the His-Purkinjé network network serves as a structural substrate for the observed broad band spectrum (Goldberger et al., 1985) (cf. Figure 2.4.3). Babloyantz and Destexhe (1988) construct the power spectrum of a four minute record of ECG which also shows a broad band structure (Figure 4.4.5) which can arise from stochastic or deterministic processes. Unlike the power-law spectra found for the single QRS complex, Babloyantz and Destexhe find an exponential power spectrum. The exponential form has been observed in a number of chaotic systems and has been used to characterize deterministic chaos by a number of authors (Greenside, Ahlers, Hohenberg and Walden, 1982; Sigeti and Horsthemke, 1987). This in itself is rather difficult to make consonant with the correlation dimension of Grassberger and Procaccia:

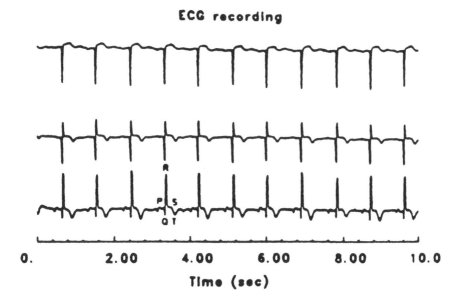

Figure 4.4.4. ECG recording of a normal human heart. The signal is digitized at regular time intervals such as to obtain a set of N points forming the time series (sampling frequency of 250 Hz with 12 bit resolution and 4th order low pass filters were used) (from Babloyantz and Destexhe, 1980 with permission).

218

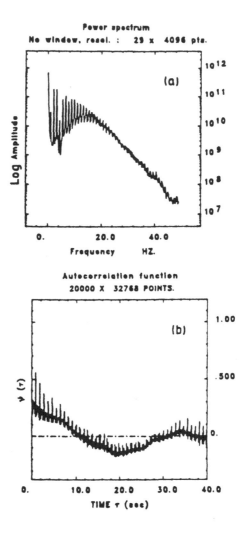

Figure 4.4.5. (a) Semi-logarithmic plot of a power spectrum from ECG showing
exponential decay at high frequencies followed by a flat region at still
higher frequencies (not shown). The flat region accounts for instrumental
noise. (b) The time decay of the autocorrelation function is characteristic
of aperiodic dynamics (from Babloyantz and Destexhe, 1988 with permission).

$$C(r) \sim r^{\nu} \tag{4.4.2}$$

since by the Tauberian Theorem (4.4.2) implies that for small r the corresponding correlation function is

$$S(\omega) \sim \frac{1}{\omega^{\nu+1}} \tag{4.4.3}$$

for large ω. Whereas if the power spectrum is exponential

$$S(\omega) \sim e^{-\gamma\omega} \tag{4.4.4}$$

then the corresponding correlation function is

$$C(r) \sim \frac{\gamma}{\gamma^2 + r^2} \quad . \tag{4.4.5}$$

Thus it would seem that the cardiac time series is not fractal, but further measures establish that it is in fact chaotic.

A phase portrait of the ECG attractor may be constructed from the time series using Taken's reconstruction theorem. Figure 4.4.6 depicts such a portrait in three-dimensional phase space using two different delay times. The two phase portraits look different; however, their topological properties are identical. It is clear that these portraits depict an attractor unlike the closed curves of a limit cycle describing periodic dynamics. Further evidence for this is obtained by calculating the correlational dimension using the Grassberger Procaccia correlation function; this dimension is found to range from 3.5 to 5.2 using 4-minute segments of data or 6×10^4 points.

The successive intersection of the trajectory with a plane located at Q in Figure 4.4.6 constitutes a Poincaré surface of section. In Figure 4.4.7 we see a return map between successive points of intersection, i.e.,the set of points $P_0, \ldots, P_N$ are related by $P_n = f(P_{n-1})$, where f is the return map. This obvious noninvertible functional relationship between these points indicates the presence of a deterministic chaotic dynamics (cf. Figure 4.4.7b). Babloyantz and Destexhe (1988) qualify this result by pointing out that because of the high dimensionality of the cardiac attractor, no coherent functional relationships between successive points were observed in other Poincaré surfaces of section, however, correlational dimensions were calculated for a total of 36 phase portraits and yielded the results quoted previously, i.e.,the correlation dimension spans the interval 3.6 ± 0.01 to 5.2 ± 0.01.

220

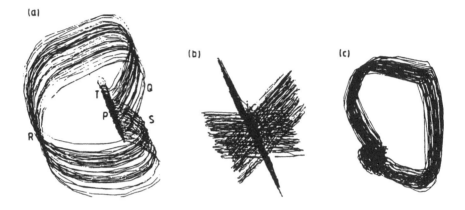

Figure 4.4.6. Phase portraits of human ECG constructed in three-dimensional space. A two-dimensional projection is displayed for two values of the delay τ: (a) 12 ms and (b) 1200 ms. (c) represents the phase portrait constructed form the three simultaneous leads of Figure 4.4.4. These portraits are far from the single closed curve which would describe a periodic activity (from Babloyantz and Destexhe, 1988 with permission).

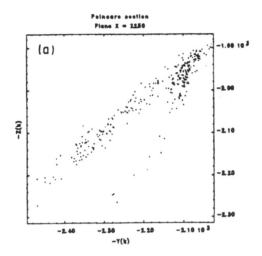

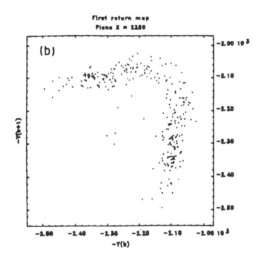

Figure 4.4.7. The Poincaré map of normal heart activity. Intersection of the phase portrait with $Y-Z$ plane $(X =$const$)$ in the region Q of Figure 4.4.6. First
return map constructed form the Y-coordinate of the previous section. We
see that there may be a simple noninvertible relationship between successive intersections (from Babloyantz and Destexhe, 1988 with permission).

222

Another indicator that the normal sinus rhythm is not strictly periodic is the broad band $1/f$-like spectrum observed by the analysis of interbeat interval variations in healthy subjects (Kobayashi and Musha, 1982; Goldberger et al., 1985). The heart rate is modulated by a complicated combination of respiratory, sympathetic and parasympathetic regulators. Akselrod, Gordon, Ubel, Shannon, Barger and Cohen (1981) showed that suppression of these effects considerably alters the $R-R$ interval power spectrum in healthy individuals, but a broad band spectrum persists. Using the interbeat sequence as a discrete time series Babloyantz and Destexhe evaluated the correlation dimension of $R-R$ intervals to be 5.9 ± 0.4 with typically 1000 intervals in the series. This dimension is significantly higher than that of the overall ECG, but we do not as yet understand the relation in the dynamics of the two quantities.

Babloyantz and Destexhe (1988) arrive at the conclusion reached earlier by Goldberger et al. (1985) among others that the normal human heart follows deterministic dynamics of a chaotic nature. The unexpected aspect of the present results are the high dimensions of the chaotic attractors. In any event there is no way that the "conventional wisdom" of the ECG consisting of periodic oscillations can be maintained in light of these new results.

4.5   The Electroencephalogram Data and the Reconstruction Technique

It has been well over a century since it was discovered that the mammalian brain generates a small but measurable electrical signal. The electroencephalograms (EEG) of small animals were measured by Caton in 1875, and in man by Berger in 1925. It had been thought by the mathematician N. Wiener, among others, that *generalized harmonic analysis* would provide the mathematical tools necessary to penetrate the mysterious relations between the EEG time series and the functioning of the brain. The progress along this path has been slow however, and the understanding and interpretation of EEG's remains quite elusive. After 112 years one can only determine intermittent correlations between the activity of the brain and that found on EEG records. There is no taxonomy of EEG patterns which delineates the correspondence between those patterns and brain activity. The clinical interpretation of EEG records is made by a complex process of visual pattern recognition and association on the part of the clinician, and significantly less often through the use of Fourier transforms. To some degree the latter technique is less useful than it might be because most EEG centers are not equipped with the computers necessary for detailed analysis of the time series.

The electroencephalographic signal is obtained from a number of standard contact configurations of electrodes attached by conductive paste to the scalp. The actual signal is in the microvolt range and must be amplified several orders of magnitude before it is recorded. Layne, Mayer-Kress and Holzfuss (1986) emphasize that the EEG is a weak signal in a sea of noise so that the importance of skilled electrode placement and inspection for artifacts of the recording protocol cannot be over estimated (Hanley, 1984). Note that pronounced artifacts often originate from slight movements of the electrodes and from contraction of muscles below the electrodes.

As we have mentioned, the relationship between the neural physiology of the brain and the overall electrical signal measured at the brain's surface is not understood. In Figure 4.5.1 is depicted the complex ramified structure of typical nerve cells in the cerebral cortex (note its similarity to the fractal structures discussed in Chapter 2). The electrical signals originate from the interconnections of the neurons through collections of dendritic tendrils interleaving the brain mass. These collections of dendrites generate signals that are correlated in space and time near the surface of the brain, and their propagation from one region of the brain's surface to another can actually be followed in real time. This signal is attenuated by the skull and scalp before it is measured by the EEG contacts.

The long standing use of Fourier decomposition in the analysis of EEG time series has provided ample opportunity to attribute significance to a number of frequency intervals in the EEG power spectrum. The power associated with the EEG signal is essentially the mean square voltage at a particular frequency. The power is distributed over the frequency interval 0.5 to 100 Hz, with most of it concentrated in the interval 1 to 30 Hz. This range is further subdivided into four sub-intervals, for historical rather than clinical reasons: the *delta*, 1-3 Hz; the *theta*, 4-7 Hz; the *alpha*, 8-14 Hz; and the *beta* for frequencies above 14 Hz. Certain of these frequencies dominate in different states of awareness. A typical EEG signal looks like a random time series with contributions from throughout the spectrum appearing with random phases. This aperiodic signal changes throughout the day and changes clinically with sleep, i.e., its high frequency random content appears to attenuate with sleep, leaving an *alpha* rhythm dominating the EEG signal. The erratic behavior of the signal is so robust that it persists, as pointed out by Freeman

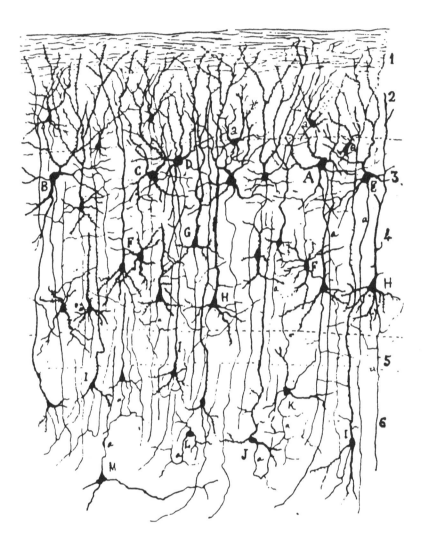

Figure 4.5.1. The complex ramified structure of typical nerve cells in the cerebral cortex is depicted.

(1987), through all but the most drastic situations including near-lethal levels of anesthesia, several minutes of asphyxia, or the complete surgical isolation of a slab of cortex. The random aspect of the signal is more than apparent, in particular, the olfactory EEG has a Gaussian amplitude histogram, a rapidly attenuating autocorrelation function, and a broad spectrum that resembles "1/f noise" (Freeman, 1975).

In this section we intend to review the applications of the embedding theorem to EEG time series obtained under a variety of clinical situations. This application will enable us to construct measures of the degree of irregularity of the time series, such as the correlation and information dimensions. We also briefly review Freeman's neural net model of the olfactory system of a rat.

In Section 4.5.2 we compare a number of these measures applied to EEG times series from a brain undergoing epileptic seizure with those of normal brain activity (cf. Figure 4.5.2). A clear reduction in the dimensionality of the time series is measured for a brain in seizure as compared with normal activity. In addition to the processing of human EEG seizure data by Babloyantz and Destexhe (1988) the application of the neural net model by Freeman to model induced seizures in rats is reviewed. A clear correlation between the measure of the degree of irregularity of the EEG signal and the activity state of the brain is observed.

4.5.1 Normal brain activity

Because of its pervasiveness it probably bears repeating that the traditional methods of analyzing EEG time series rely of the paradigm that all temporal variations are decomposable into harmonic and periodic vibrations. The reconstruction technique, however, reinterprets the time series as a multidimensional geometrical object generated by a deterministic dynamical process which is not necessarily a superposition of periodic oscillations. If the dynamics are reducible to deterministic laws, then the phase portraits of the system converge toward a finite subset of phase space. This invariant subset is the attractor. Thus the phase space trajectories constructed from the data should be confined to lie along such an attractor. In Figure 4.5.3 is depicted the projection of the EEG attractor onto a two-dimensional subspace for two different pairs of leads using different segments of the corresponding time series.

226

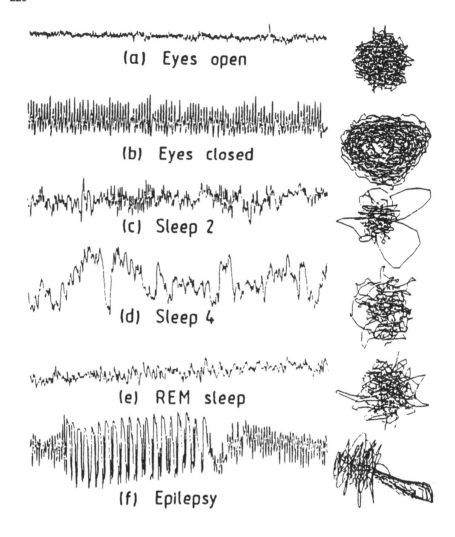

Figure 4.5.2. Typical episodes of the electrical activity of the human brain as recorded from the electroencephalogram (EEG) together with the corresponding phase portraits. These portraits are the two-dimensional projections of three-dimensional constructions. The EEG was recorded on a FM analog tape and processed off-line (signal digitized in 12 bits, 250 Hz frequency, 4th order 120 Hz low pass filter) (from Babloyantz and Destexhe, 1987 with permission).

C3-T3 Awake but quiet

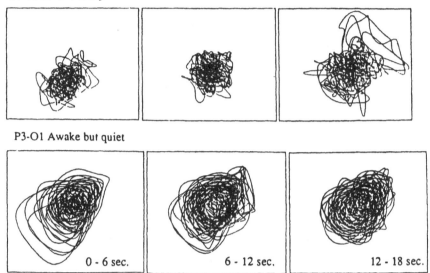

P3-O1 Awake but quiet

0 - 6 sec.   6 - 12 sec.   12 - 18 sec.

Figure 4.5.3.   Two-dimensional phase portraits, $V(t_k + \Delta T)$vs$V(t_k)$, of EEG data. Each portrait is generated by 3000 data points and consecutive portraits (in time) appear from left to right (from Mayer-Kress and Layne, 1987 with permission).

Using the probe positions depicted in Figure 4.5.4, Mayer-Kress and Layne use the reconstruction technique on the EEG time series to obtain the phase portraits in Figure 4.5.3. These phase portraits do suggest chaotic attractors with diverging trajectories, however, the EEG time series seems to be *nonstationary*. That is to say that the average position of the time series defined over some time interval that is long compared with most of the EEG activity, is observed to change on a longer time scale. Also the EEG trajectory is seen to undergo large excursions in the phase space at odd times. From this Layne et al. (1986) conclude that the EEG time series are nonstationary and of high dimension, in which case the concepts of "attractor" and "fractal dimension" do not apply, since these are asymptotic or stationary properties of a dynamic system. Babloyantz and Destexhe (1987) point out that this nonstationarity is strictly true for awake states, however it appears that stationarity can be found in the time series from patients that are sleeping and from those having certain pathologies.

Following Farmer, Ott and York (1983), Layne et al. (1986) use a slightly different weighting than (3.3.5):

$$C_m(r) = \lim_{M \to \infty} \frac{1}{M_{ref}} \sum_{i=1}^{M_{ref}} \frac{1}{M} \sum_{j=1}^{M} \Theta\left[r - |\mathbf{X}_i - \mathbf{X}_j|\right] \qquad (4.5.1)$$

where M_{ref} is the number of references points used in the calculation. We see here that not all pairs of points are averaged in (4.5.1), but rather 200 equally spaced reference points in the "attractor" are averaged over. There are typically 2×10^4 data points, so that using the original method would require far too much time even on a CRAY-XMP computer to include all possible pairs of points. They average over 200 reference points because $C_m(r)$ is sensitive to the local structure of the "attractor" i.e., certain region of the "attractor" are visited more often than others and are therefore more important.

In Figure 4.5.5 *log* $C_m(r)$ versus *log r* is shown for an embedding dimension $m = 20$ with typical EEG data. Again one can determine a "dimension" by fitting the region $-2 \leq log\ r \leq -1$. Mayer-Kress and Layne (1987) introduce the term (dimensional) complexity parameter to emphasize caution in the application of this technique to EEG time series data. In Figure 4.5.6 the variation in the measured dimension from the local slope is depicted versus *log r*. The local slope is determined by a weighted least squares fit of a tangent vector to each value for *log r*. Note that the error is of the same

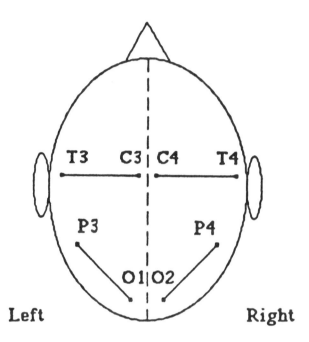

Figure 4.5.4.   Two standard EEG leads from the international 10-20 systems.

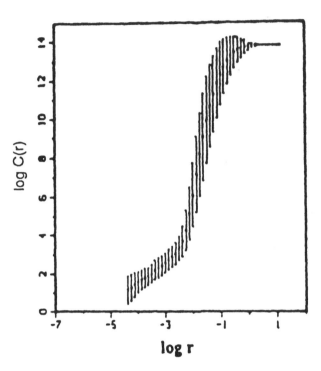

Figure 4.5.5. Dimension curve, with embedding dimension $N = 20$, for typical EEG data. This calculation is based on 15000 data points k (30 seconds of data) and 200 reference points. Error bars indicate standard deviations in the distribution of the average number of vectors N at distance r. Figures 4.5.5 through 4.5.7 are from the same awake but quite EEG data (lead T3-C3) (from Mayer-Kress and Layne, 1987 with permission).

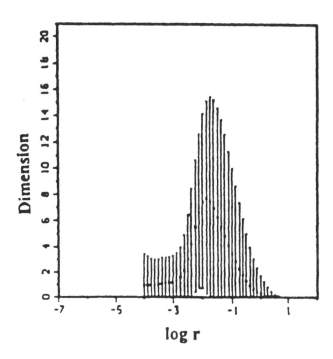

Figure 4.5.6. Local slope d of the "dimension" curve versus $\log r$. Note the asymptotic values of $d = 1$ for $r \to \infty$ and $d = 0$ (from Mayer-Kress and Layne, 1987 with permission).

order of magnitude as the dimension itself and this effect seems to increase with embedding dimension. In Figure 4.5.7 we see that the dimension does not saturate with increasing embedding dimension, Babloyantz and Destexhe (1986) observed rather high dimensions for awake patients or those in REM sleep and cautioned that the Grassberger-Procaccia correlation diversion may not be meaningful at these large values. Mayer-Kress and Layne (1987) comment:

> "Even though we are unable to calculate the 'actual dimension' of EEG, we believe that our numerical results reveal a comparative difference between two states of consciousness, i.e., awake but quiet, and general anesthesia."

It should be emphasized that the large error bars depicted in Figure 4.5.6 and 4.5.7 call into question the idea of using the Grassberger-Procaccia correlation dimension to characterize EEG time series. However, it is the choice of algorithm that determines how "accurately" the correlation dimension is determined. The pessimism voiced by Mayer-Kress and Layn (1987) for the utility of this concept is not shared by a large regiment of the nonlinear dynamics community, but their cautionary remarks have helped to stimulate the development of a number of alternative and more efficient numerical algorithms to evaluate $C_m(r)$.

The brain wave activity of an individual during various stages of sleep was analyzed by Babloyantz (1986). She uses the standard division of sleeping into four stages. In stage one, the individual drifts in and out of sleep. In stage two, the slightest noise will arouse the sleeper, whereas in stage three a loud noise is required. The final stage is one of deep sleep. This is the normal first sequence of stages one goes through during a sleep cycle. Afterwards the cycle is reversed back through stages three and two at which time dreams set in and the individual manifests rapid eye movement (REM). The dream state is followed by stage two after which the initial sequence begins again. The EEG phase portraits for each of these stages of sleep are depicted in Figure 4.5.8. It is clear that whatever the form of the attractor it is not static, that is to say, it varies with the level of sleep. Correspondingly, the correlational dimension calculated using (4.5.1) yields decreasing values as sleep deepens.

In Table 4.5.1 is summarized a number of dimension calculations for EEG time series for various states of brain activity obtained by a number of investigators. Using these results Mayer-Kress and Layne (1987) reached the following conclusions:

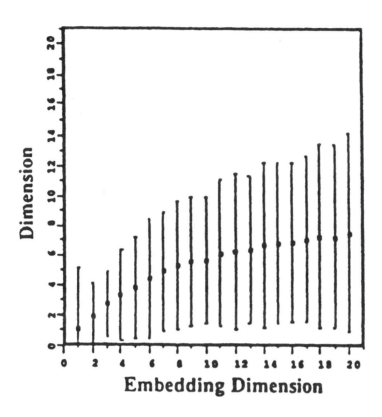

Figure 4.5.7. Observed "dimension" as a function of embedding dimension N. Dimension values at each m were calculated by a weighted least squares fit. The length of the line segments L for each fit ranged from 7 to 9 unit divisions in $\log r$ on the "dimension curve" (from Mayer-Kress and Layne, 1987 with permission).

234

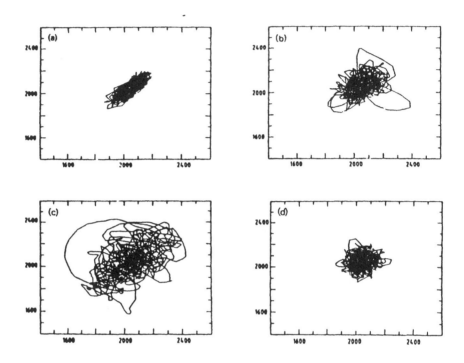

Figure 4.5.8. Two-dimensional phase portraits derived from the EEG of (a) an awake
subject, (b) sleep stage two, (c) sleep stage four, (d) REM sleep. The time
series $x_0(t)$ is made of $N = 4000$ equidistant points. The central EEG
derivation C4-A1 according to the Jasper system. Recorded with PDP
11-44, 100 Hz for 40 s. The value of the shift from 1s to 1d is $r = 10\Delta t$
(from Babloyantz, 1986 with permission).

Table 4.5.1. Chaos in the Brain

The data in this table have been contributed by a number of authors and is published in Mayer-Kress and Layne (1987). The "dimension" of the EEG's are calculated under a number of different conditions, i.e., changes in the processing as well as cognitive parameters.

State of the Brain	Lead	Sampling Rate (Hz)	Delay τ(msec)	Total Time (sec)	Maximal Embedding Dimension	Dimension
Albano et al. (1987)						
Quiet, awake,	?	500	10	5.8	19	eyes closed 2.6 ± 0.2
Quiet, awake, eyes open	?	500	6	5.8	19	∞
Babloyantz et al. (1985, 1986)						
Quiet, awake	C4-A1	100	100	40	10	6.1 ± 0.05
Sleep stage 2	C4-A1	100	100	40	6	5.0 ± 0.1
Sleep stage 4	C4-A1	100	100	40	5	4.1 ± 0.1
REM sleep	C4-A1	100	100	40	10	8.2 ± 0.04
Petit mal seizure	?	1200	15.8	5	7	2.05 ± 0.09
Mayer-Kress & Layne (1987)[†]						
Quiet, awake	P3-01	100-500	10-40	10-30	20	4-7 ± 3-5
Quiet, awake	P4-02	100-500	10-40	10-30	20	4-7 ± 3-5
Quiet, awake	C3-T3	100-500	10-40	10-30	20	7-8 ± 5
Quiet, awake	C4-T4	100-500	10-40	10-30	20	7-8 ± 5

[†]Data from J. Hanley

236

"(1) The 'fractal dimension' of the EEG cannot be determined regionally, due to non-stationarity of the signal and subsequent limitations in the amount of acceptable data."

"(2) EEG data must be analyzed in a comparative sense with the subject acting as their control."

"(3) In a few cases (awake but quiet, eyes closed) with limited time samples, it appears that the dimension algorithm converge to finite values."

"(4) Dimension analysis and attractor reconstruction could prove to be useful tools for examining the EEG and complement the more classical methods based on spectral properties."

"(5) Besides being a useful tool in determining the optimal delay-time for dimension calculations, the mutual information content is a quantity which is sensitive to different brain states."

It is also clear from this table that it is the results for the awake state that calls into question the fractal dimension of the EEG time series. These conclusions are consistent with those of Babloyantz and Destexhe (1987) and Albano et al. (1987).

The data processing results are strongly suggestive of the existence of chaotic attractors determining the dynamics of brain activity underlying the observed EEG signals. This interpretation of the data would be strongly supported by the existence of mathematical models that could reproduce the observed behavior; such as in the examples shown earlier in this chapter. One such model has been developed by Freeman (1987) to describe the dynamics of the olfactory system, consisting of the olfactory bulb (OB), anterior nucleus (AON) and prepyriform cortex (PC). Each segment consists of a collection of excitatory or inhibitory neurons which in isolation is modeled by a nonlinear second order ordinary differential equation. The basal olfactory EEG is not sinusoidal as one might have expected, but is irregular and aperiodic. This intrinsic unpredictability is manifest in the approach to zero of the autocorrelation function of the time series data. This behavior is captured in Freeman's dynamic model.

The model of Freeman generates a voltage time series from sets of coupled nonlinear differential equations with interconnections that are specified by the anatomy of the olfactory bulb, the anterior nucleus and the prepyriform cortex. The neurons in each collection simultaneously perform four serial operations: "(1) nonlinear conversion of afferent axonal impulses to dendritic currents; (2) linear spatiotemporal integration; (3) nonlinear conversion of summed dendritic current to a pulse density and (4) linear axonal delay, temporal dispersion, translation and spatial divergence.'' The operation of the basic integrator in the model consists of two distinct parts: a linear time dependent operator

$$F(V_n) \equiv \frac{1}{ab} \frac{d^2}{dt^2} V_n(t) + \left[\frac{1}{a} + \frac{1}{b}\right] \frac{dV_n(t)}{dt} + \frac{1}{ab} V_n(t) \qquad (4.5.2)$$

and a nonlinear time-invariant part $G(V)$. Here $V(t)$ denotes the instantaneous voltage and the subscript n denotes the particular collection of neurons to which it belongs. The rate parameters are fit to data to yield $a = 220/\text{sec}$ and $b = 720/\text{sec}$. The equation for the nonlinear part of the input voltage (V) and the output variable P are;

$$Q = \begin{cases} Q_m(1 - \exp[-(e^V - 1)/Q_m]) & , \quad V > -u_0 \\ -1 & , \quad V \le -u_0 \end{cases} \qquad (4.5.3)$$

where

$$u_0 = -\ln\left[1 - Q_m \ln(1 + 1/Q_m)\right] \qquad (4.5.4)$$

and

$$P = u_0(Q + 1) \qquad (4.5.5)$$

with $Q_m = 5.0$ is the asymptote of the sigmoidal curve depicted in Figure 4.5.9. The voltage dependent gain is

$$\frac{dP}{dV} = u_0 \exp\left\{V - (e^V - 1)/Q_m\right\} \qquad (4.5.6)$$

where

$$V_{max} = \ln Q_m \qquad (4.5.7)$$

and the displacement of the maximal gain to the right increases with increasing Q_m, a critical property of the mechanism.

Subsets of equations are formed by taking two of the basic integrators and coupling them through feedback relations indexed by e. A second type of subset indexed by i is formed with these feedback relations if the output voltage of each is inverted before inputed to the other. Each output is multiplied by a gain coefficient k_{lj} where $V_j = k_{lj}P_l$ and $0.2 < k_{lj} < 2.0$ to optimize stability and sensitivity. Four types of internal connections are identified: k_{ee}, k_{ei}, k_{ie} and k_{ii} so that the equations for the connected subsets take the form

238

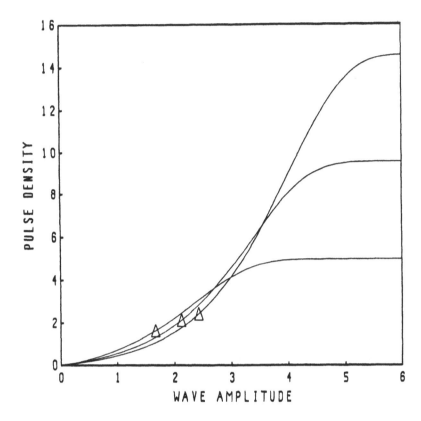

Figure 4.5.9. Sigmoid curves representing the non-linear relation between axonal firing
rates (ordinate) and dendritic current (abscissa) at trigger zones of OB and
PC neurons. The curve was derived in part from the Hodgkin-Huxley
equations. It was evaluated by fitting it to measurements of the normalized probability of firing of OB and PC neurons conditional on the amplitude and time of occurrence of the EEG. The set of curves shows 3 levels
of background, steadystate activity (triangles), reflecting the change in the
curve with increasing motivation from rest (lowest curve). The sigmoidal
shape of the curve reflects mechanisms that are of major importance for
stabilizing normal brain function (from Freeman, 1986 with permission).

$$F(V_{e1,j}) = k_{ee} \ P_{e2,j} - k_{ie}(P_{i1,j} + P_{i2,j}) + k_{ee} \sum_{k \neq j}^{N} P_{e1,k} + I_j \qquad (4.5.8)$$

$$F(V_{e2,j}) = k_{ee} P_{e1,j} - k_{ie} P_{i1,j} \qquad (4.5.9)$$

$$F(V_{i2,j}) = k_{ei} P_{e1,j} - k_{ii} P_{i1,j} \qquad (4.5.10)$$

$$F(V_{i1,j}) = k_{ei}(P_{e1,j} + P_{e2,j}) - k_{ii} P_{i2,j} + k_{ii} \sum_{k \neq j}^{N} P_{i1,k} \quad , \qquad (4.5.11)$$

where I_j is the output of the jth subset.

When an arbitrarily small input pulse is received at the receptor, the model system generates continuing activity that has the statistical properties of the background EEG of resting animals. A comparison of the model output is compared with that of a rat in Figure 4.5.10. Freeman (1987) comments:

"Close visual inspection of resting EEG's and their simulations show that they are not indistinguishable, but statistical procedures by which to describe their differences have not yet been devised. Both appear to be chaotic on the basis of the properties listed, but the forms of their chaotic attractors and their dimensions have not yet been derived."

The utility of chaotic activity in natural systems have by now been pointed out by a number of scientists, there being four or five categories depending on one's discipline. In the olfactory neural context Freeman (1987) points out that chaos provides a rapid and unbiased access to any member of a collection of latent attractors, any of which may be selected at random on any inhalation depending on the olfactory environment. He goes on to say:

"The low-dimensional 'noise' is 'turned off' at the moment of bifurcation to a patterned attractor, and it is 'turned on' again on reverse bifurcation as the patterned attractor vanishes. Second, the chaotic attractor provides for global and continuous spatiotemporally unstructured neural activity, which is essential to maintain neurons in optimal condition by preventing atrophy of disuse in periods of low olfactory demand. Third, one of the patterned attractors provides for responding to the background or contextual odor complex. It appears that a novel odor interferes with the background and leads to failure of convergence to any patterned attractor, and that chaotic OB output may then serve by default to signal to the *PC the presence of a significant but unidentified departure form the environmental status quo detected by the receptors.* The correct classification of a novel order by this scheme can occur as rapidly and reliably as the classification of any known odor, without requiring an exhaustive search through an ensemble of classifiable patterns that is stored in the brain. Fourth,

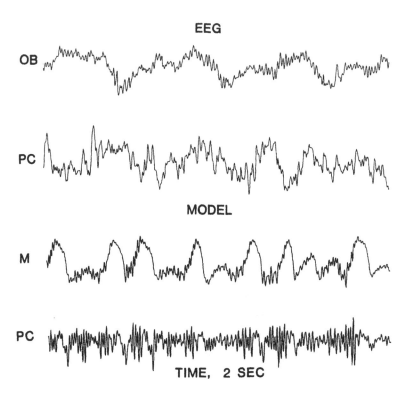

Figure 4.5.10.   Examples of chaotic background activity generated by the model, simu-
                 lating bulbar unit activity and the EEGs of the OB, AON and PC.
                 $Q_m = 5.0$, $K_{ME} = 1.5$, $K_{EG} = 0.67$, $K_{EP} = 1.0$, $K_{PM} = 0.1$, $K_{MA} = 1$,
                 $K_{EA} = 1.5$, $K_{AI} = 1.0$, $K_{AP} = 1$. The *top two traces* are representative
                 records of the OB and PC EEGs from a rat at rest breathing through
                 the nose (from Freeman, 1986 with permission).

the chaotic activity evoked by a novel odor provides unstructured activity that can drive the formation of a new nerve cell assembly by strengthening of synapses between pairs of neurons having highly correlated activity (the Hebb rule in its differential form). Thereby chaos allows the system to escape from its established repertoire of responses in order to add a new response to a novel stimulus under reinforcement.''

These speculations have been narrowly focused on the dynamics of the olfactory system, but they are easily generalizable to a much broader neuronal context. For example we have noted elsewhere in this monograph how chaos may be an integral part of the learning process. It has also appeared that the dynamics in other complex systems manifest chaos in order to ensure adaptability of the underlying process. Conrad (1986) denotes five possible functional roles for chaos. The first is the generation of diversity as in the prey-predator species where the exploratory behavior of the animal is enhanced. The second is the preservation of diversity in which the diversity of behavior is used by the prey to act unpredictably and thereby elude being the supper for the predator. The third possible role of chaos is maintenance of adaptability that is to disentrain processes. In populations this would correspond to keeping a broad age spectrum. The fourth is the interaction between population dynamics and gene structure (cross-level effects). Chaos on the genetic level would contribute to the diversity and adaptability on the population level. Finally, the dissipation of disturbances is achieved by the sensitivity of orbits on the chaotic attractor to initial conditions. In this way the attractor acts as a heat bath for the system and ensures its stability.

4.5.2 Epilepsy, the reduced dimension

One of the more dramatic results that has been obtained in recent years has to do with the relative degree of order in the electrical activity of the human cortex in an epileptic human patient and in normal persons engaged in various activities (cf. Figure 4.5.2). Babloyantz and Destexhe (1986) used an EEG time series from a human patient undergoing a ''petit mal'' seizure to demonstrate the dramatic change in the neural chaotic attractor using the phase space reconstruction technique. Freeman (1986) has induced an epileptic form seizure in the prepyriform cortex of cat, rat and rabbit. The seizures closely resembles variants of psychomotor or petit mal epilepsy in humans. His dynamic model, discussed in the preceding section, enables him to propose neural mechanisms for the seizures, and investigate the model structure of the chaotic attractor in transition from the normal to the seizure state. As we have discussed, the attractor is a direct consequence of the deterministic nature of brain activity, and what distinguishes normal activity from that observed during epileptic seizures is a sudden drop in the dimensionality of the attractor. Babloyantz and Destexhe (1986) determine the dimensionality of the brain's attractor to be 4.05 ± 0.5 in deep sleep and to have the much lower dimensionality of 2.05 ± 0.09 in the epileptic state.

Epileptic seizures are manifestations of a characteristic state of brain activity that can and often does occur without apparent warning. The spontaneous transition of the brain from a normal state to a epileptic state may be induced by various means, but is usually the result of functional disorders or lesions. Such a seizure manifests an abrupt, violent, usually self-terminating disorder of the cortex. One can think of it as an instability induced by the breakdown of neural mechanisms that ordinarily maintain the normal state of the cortex and thereby assure its stability. In the previous section we argued that there is evidence to indicate that the normal state is described by a chaotic attractor. We now find that the seizure state is also a chaotic attractor, but with a lower dimension. Babloyantz and Destexhe (1986) were concerned with seizures of short duration (approximately five seconds in length) known as "petit mal." This type of generalized epilepsy may invade the entire cerebral cortex and shows a bilateral symmetry between the left and right hemispheres. As is apparent in the EEG time series in Figure 4.5.11 there is a sharp transition from the apparently noisy normal state to the organized, apparently periodic epileptic state. The transition from the epileptic state back to the normal state is equally sharp.

A sequence of stimulations applied to the lateral olfactory tract (LOT) will induce seizures when the ratio of background activity to induced activity exceeds a critical value (Freeman, 1986). In Figure 4.5.12 the regular spike train of the seizure induced by the applied stimulation shown at the left is depicted. These data are used to define the phase space variables $\{x_0(t), x_0(t + \tau), \ldots, x_0[t + (m - 1)\tau]\}$ necessary to construct the phase portrait of the system in both normal and epileptic states.

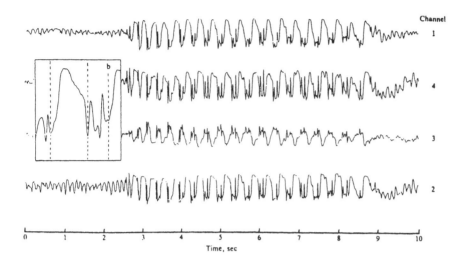

Figure 4.5.11.   (a) EEG recording of a human epileptic seizure of petit mal activity. Channel 1 (left) and channel 3 (right) measure the potential differences between frontal and parietal regions of the scalp, whereas channel 2 (left) and channel 4 (right) correspond to the measures between vertex and temporal regions. This seizure episode, lasting 5 seconds is the longest and the least noise-contaminated EEG selected from a 24-hr recording on a magnetic tape of a single patient. Digital PDP 11 equipment was used. The signal was filtered below 0.2 Hz and above 45 Hz and is sampled in 12 bits at 1200 Hz. (b) One pseudocycle is formed from a relaxation wave. (From Babloyantz and Destexhe, 1986 with permission.)

244

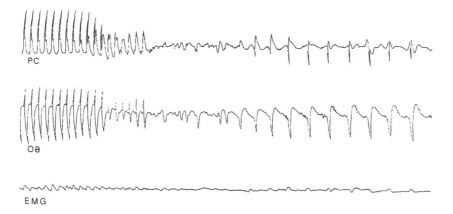

Figure 4.5.12.   The last 1.7 s is shown of a 3-s pulse train to the LOT (10 V, 0.08 ms,
                  10/s), with decrement in response amplitudes begining at 0.7 s before
                  the end of the train. Seizure spike trains begin uncoordinated in both
                  structures and settle into a repetitive train at 3.4/s with the PC spike
                  leading by 25 ms both the OB spike and EMG spike from the ipsilateral
                  temporal muscle (from Freeman, 1986 with permission).

In Figure 4.5.13 is depicted the projection of the epileptic attractor onto a two-dimensional subspace for four different angles of observation. Babloyantz and Destexhe (1986) point out that the structure of this attractor is reminiscent of the spiral or screw chaotic attractor of Rössler (1979). Freeman (1986) did not associate the attractor he observed with any of the canonical forms, but he was able to capture a number of the qualitative features of the dynamics with calculations using his model. It is clear in Figure 4.5.14 that the attractor for a rat during seizures is well captured by the model dynamics. He acknowledged that the unpredictability in the detail of the simulated and recorded seizure spike trains indicate that they are chaotic, and in this regard agree with the conclusion of Babloyantz and Destexhe. Note the similarity in the attractor depicted in Figure 4.5.14 with that for the heart in Figure 4.4.6c. Let us see how the latter authors calculated the dimension of the reconstructed attractor using the limited data sample available in the single realization of human epileptic seizure.

In Figure 4.5.15 is recorded the $log\ C_m(r)$ versus $log\ r$ epileptic data for six values of m. If $C(r) \sim r^v$ we would expect a straight line in this plot, with slope v. In practice, however, the line will never be perfectly straight for all $log\ r$ because of the finite size of the vectors in the multi-dimensional reconstruction. There is usually a smaller region over which a straight line may be fitted, and a dimension calculated. It is difficult to say if the "dimension" determined from this limited domain is significant or not.

In Figure 4.5.16 these results are used to determine the dependence of the correlation dimension on the embedding dimension and are compared with the white noise results. We see here a clear indication that the epileptic state possesses a chaotic attractor and therefore should have a deterministic dynamic representation in either three of four variables. The low dimensionality of the attractor is indicative of the extreme coherence of the brain during an epileptic seizure relative to normal brain activity.

In Section 4.2 we discussed how certain neural activity could be modeled by a chaotic attractor. It is possible to speculate that such chaotic neural activity could be benign or even beneficial. Rapp et al. (1987) point out the possible utility of such neural activity in searching memory and in the early stages of decision making. The arguments rest on the recent quantitative results in control theory which illustrate how certain

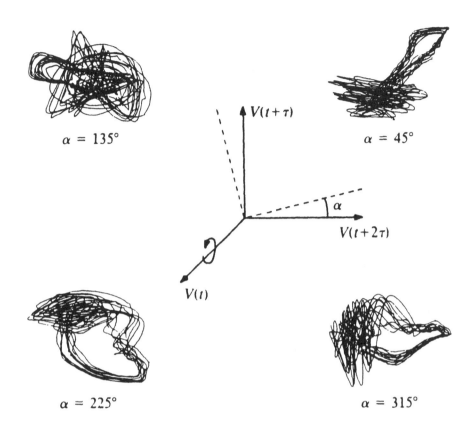

Figure 4.5.13.   Phase portraits of human epileptic seizure. First, the attractor is
represented in a three-dimensional phase space. The figure shows two-
dimensional projections after a rotation of an angle α around the $V(t)$
axis. The time series is constructed from the first channel of figure 1
($n = 5000$ equidistant points and $\tau = 19\Delta t$). Nearly identical phase portraits are found for all τ in the range from $17\Delta t$ to $25\Delta t$ and also in
other instances of seizure (from Babloyantz and Destexhe, 1986 with
permission).

247

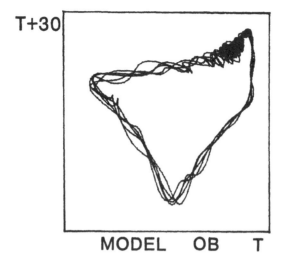

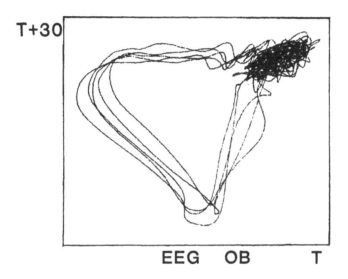

Figure 4.5.14. Comparison of the output of the trace from granule cells (G) in the model (above) with the OB seizure from a rat (below), each plotted against itself lagged 30 ms in time. Duration is 1.0 s; rotation is counterclockwise (from Freeman, 1986 with permission).

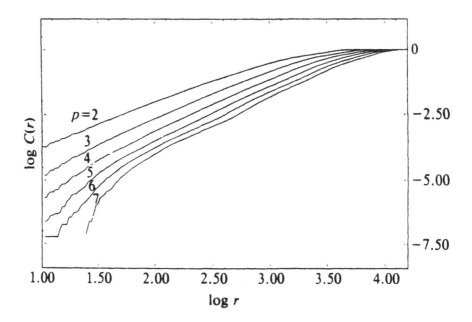

Figure 4.5.15.   The logarithm of the correlation integral is plotted versus that of the separation r, $M = 6 \times 10^3$ and $\tau = 19\Delta t$ (from Babloyantz and Destexhe, 1986 with permission).

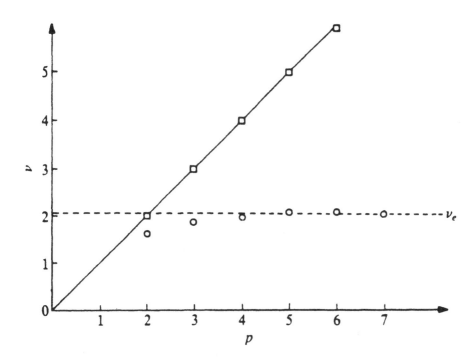

Figure 4.5.16. Dependence of the correlation dimension ν on the embedding dimension N for a white noise signal (□) and for the epileptic attractor (○)
with $\tau = 19\Delta t$. The saturation toward a value ν is the manisfestation of
a deterministic dynamics (from Babloyantz and Destexhe, 1988 with
permission).

complex systems can be functionally optimized through the introduction of noise (Kolata, 1984). On the other hand, most efforts have focused on the deleterious effects of chaos, see e.g. the notion of dynamic diseases, Mackey and Glass (1977), in particular the possible relationship between neural chaos and failures of neural regulation. There have been a number of suggestions on the possible role for chaos in epileptogenesis (see Rapp et al. (1987) for a list of references). The latter authors make the point that because of the decrease in dimensionality that a seizure may not itself be chaotic, i.e., there is a decrease in the disorder of the brain activity. "The seizure might serve as a corrective resynchronizing response to the loss of coherence of the brain activity that, in turn, is the result of chaotic neural behavior."

4.5.3 Task-related dimensions

The results of calculations of the degree of complexity of the EEG time series discussed in the preceding section suggests that the erratic signals from the brain are correlated with the cognitive activity of the patient. The complex electrical signal, its change in shape and amplitude are related to such states as sleep, wakefulness, alertness, problem-solving, and hearing as well as to several clinical conditions (Bullock, Orkand and Grinnel, 1981) such as epilepsy (Principe and Smith, 1982; Siegel, Grady and Miraky, 1982) and schizophrenia (Itil, 1977). This in itself is not a new result, it has been known for some time that brain activity responds in a demonstrable way to external stimulation. The direct or peripheral deterministic simulation could be electrical, optical, acoustical, etc., depending on the conditions of the experiment. This induced change in the brains' electrical activity is called an Evoked Potential. One can distinguish between an evoked potential and the spontaneous electrical activity of the brain in the following way (Chang, 1959):

"(a) It bears definite temporal relationship to the onset of the stimulus. In other words, it has definite latent period determined by the conduction distance between the point of stimulation and the point of recording. (b) It has a definite pattern of response characteristic of a specific system which is more or less predictable under similar conditions."

One strategy for understanding the dynamic behavior of the brain has been general systems analysis, or general systems theory. In this approach a system is defined as a collection of components arranged and interconnected in a definite way. As stated by Basar (1976) the components may be physical, chemical, biological or a combination of all three. From this perspective if the stimulus applied to the system is known (measured) and the response of the system to this response is known (measured) then it should be possible to estimate the properties of the system. This, of course, is not sufficient to determine all the characteristic of the "black box" but is the first step in formulating what Basar calls a "biological system analysis theory" in which special modes of thought, unique to the special nature of living systems, are required. In particular Basar points out the nonstationary nature of the spontaneous electrical activity of the brain, a property also observed by Mayer-Kress and Layne (1987) and Layne (1987) and mentioned in the preceding section.

In the general systems theory context Basar (1976) considers the analog relation of a driven relaxation oscillator and the spontaneous electrical activity of the brain. The view is not unlike the coupled bio-oscillator model of the SA and AV nodes of the heart discussed in Section 3.1, or the externally excited neurons in Section 4.2. The inappropriateness of the linear concepts of the superposition of electrical signals and the independence of different frequency modes is appreciated, and the importance of nonlinear dynamical concepts is stressed.

The brain consists of a very large population of neurons and a number of investigators have attempted to model it from the point of view of neural nets [see e.g. Basar, Flohr, Haken and Mandell (1983), and Freeman in the last section]. We will not comment further on these research activities except to point out that Basar (1983) finds a great deal in the modern development of nonlinear dynamics that is consistent with the more traditional general systems theory approach to understanding the brain through the use of evoked potentials. It is possible that the EEG time series is a consequence of pacemaker neurons in a neural population stimulating other neurons and driving them to a chaotic response, see for example the model of Freeman in the preceding section. In this way spontaneous brain activity may be a reflection of internal evoked potentials arising from endogenous brain potentials, which are seemingly due to cognitive operations of the brain. This interpretation is consistent with the results of the preceding section, i.e., the level of brain activity changes with *internal* tasks. We have not as yet associated forms to the brain response such as is done in evoked potential analysis, but that is not to say that such forms do not exist for various cognitive activities.

We have observed that in normal brain activity the visual appearance of the EEG time trace changes markedly as one changes states from quiet with eyes open, to quiet with eyes closed, through the levels of sleep to the state of rapid eye movement. In Figure 4.5.2 these changes in the time trace are obvious, but the accompanying phase space portraits are not easy to read. It might become clear after a certain amount of inspection that the attractors depicted in (c) and (d) are not so tightly constrained as those of (a) and (b), but to make this impression quantitative requires additional effort. In Table 4.5.1 the correlation dimension has been recorded for various states of the brain when it is not engaged in cognitive activity perhaps with the exception of the epileptic seizures. The dimensionality of the EEG for the simple situation of being quiet, awake, but with eyes open or closed varies from 2.6 to undetermined. Thus the absolute dimension does not seem to be a reliable indicator of the cognitive state, however, we will see that by using individuals as their own control we can reliably indicate the *changes* in their cognitive state.

In Table 4.5.2 we record the correlation dimension for one of the important applications of EEG analysis and that is anesthesia, where a reliable monitoring and control of its depth is still a problem which causes many deaths each year. Mayer-Kress and Layne (1987) determine that the "dimension" is not a sensitive indicator of the transition from light to medium anesthesia. They also find, unlike the results of Babloyantz et al. (1985, 1986) in Table 4.5.1, that there seem to be no significant changes in dimension for the various stages of natural sleep (cf. Table 4.5.3); they do find, however, that the mutual information content varies significantly with different sleep stages. Recall that following the suggestion of Fraser and Swinney (1986), Mayer-Kress and Layne (1987) use the first minimum in the mutual information content to determine the delay in the phase space reconstruction of the EEG attractor.

It is difficult to assess the significance of the dimensions found by Watt and Hameroff (1987) due to the large variances. However, the significance of the dimension of a certain excitatory anesthetic (fluroxene) seems to be better established. The dimension,

Table 4.5.2. More Chaos in the Brain

The data in this table are originally from Watt and Hameroff (1986) and Mayer-Kress
and Layne (1987). They calculate the correlation dimension of EEG time series when
the subject is under the influence of anesthesia.

State of the brain	Lead	Sampling Rate (Hz)	Delay τ (msec)	Total Time (sec)	Maximal Embedding Dimension	Dimension
Watt and Hameroff (1986)						
Quiet, awake, eyes closed	C3-P3	300	17	4	6	2.15 ± 2.0
Isoflurane anesthesia	C3-P3	300	17	4	6	2.07 ± 2.0
Thiopental anesthesia	C3-P3	300	17	4	6	1.90 ± 2.0
Mayer-Kress & Layne (1987)						
Fluroxene anesthesia	(All four)	100-500	10-40	10-30	20	8.0 ± 6.0

Table 4.5.3. Still More Chaos in the Brain

The data in this table are originally from C. Ehlers and were published and processed by Mayer-Kress and Layne (1987). They give the correlation dimension of EEG time series when the subject is completing a number of cognitive tasks. The sampling rate is 512 Hz, the delay time is in the interval 10 ms $\leq \tau \leq$ 40 ms, the total time is in the interval 10 sec $\leq$ t $\leq$ 30 sec and the maximal embedding dimension is 20.

Quiet, awake and	Lead	Dimension
Eyes closed	P3-O1	5.1 ± 5.4
Eyes closed	P4-O2	5.0 ± 4.0
Eyes open, no task	P3-O1	8.6 ± 5.1
Eyes open, no task	P4-O2	8.7 ± 5.4
Eyes closed, verbal memory	P3-O1	6.3 ± 2.9
Eyes closed, verbal memory	P4-O2	6.4 ± 3.3
Eyes closed, visual memory	P3-O1	6.1 ± 5.5
Eyes closed, abstraction	P3-O1	6.0 ± 3.4
Eyes closed, abstraction	P4-O2	6.4 ± 3.8
Eyes closed, word association	P3-O1	5.9 ± 3.5
Eyes closed, word association	P4-O2	5.5 ± 3.8
Sleep		
Onset	C3-A1	6.8 ± 6.1
Stage 4	C3-A1	5.9 ± 4.4
REM	C3-A1	6.4 ± 5.1

measured at the lead P3-O1, was reported to increase from 4.3 ± 2.2 before anesthesia to 8.0 ± 3.8 during medium fluroxene anesthesia. Further refinements of these calculations are discussed in Mayer-Kress, Yates, Benton, Deidel, Tirsch, Pöppl and Geist (1987), in which the results are shown to display a delicate dependence on details especially at high values of the dimension. The importance of all the additional analysis is the consistent finding that the dimensionality of the EEG time series increases from the normal to the anesthetized state. It should be pointed out that these errors depend on the choice of delay time τ and that perhaps a systematic study of the error to variations in τ might lead to different choices; see e.g. Babloyantz and Destexhe (1987).

Additional evidence for this conjecture is displayed in Table 4.5.3 where Mayer-Kress and Layne (1987) use the data of Ehlers to calculate the correlational dimension for a number of cognitive states. We can see a progression of the dimension magnitude from quiet, awake, eyes closed (~5) to quiet, awake, eyes closed using verbal memory (~6.3). Although with the large magnitudes of the errors it is difficult to draw definitive conclusions from these data. Notice however that the variance in dimension is decreased as the state of the brain changes from no task to one involving cognitive activity. The trend in these data seems to indicate that the dimension of the EEG time series is closely tied to the cognitive activity of the brain. Further, there is a distinct ordering of the mental task performed and the magnitude of the dimension. It would be of interest to have an independent measure of the degree of difficulty of each of these tasks. In this way we would be able to verify the conclusion suggested by the results in Table 4.5.3. This conclusion is that the lowest dimension is for the resting state of a quiet, awake subject with eyes closed, the highest dimension is for the quiet, awake subject with eyes open and the dimension increases with cognitive task difficulty.

As we mentioned, the computer has been used to process EEG time series data for quite a while and the development of the techniques for displaying computer results in a form that facilitates the interpretation of EEG records has an equally long history (Ktonas, 1983). Some of the clinical areas in which this has been done are epilepsy (Principe and Smith, 1982; Siegel et al., 1982) and schizophrenia (Itil, 1977) but as pointed out by Rapp et al. (1987) these programs have had limited effect on clinical practice. They suggest this in the case because the earlier efforts have centered on spectral analysis and its variants, and they speculate that harmonic analysis does not provide a neurologically meaningful measure of brain electrical activity. They rightly point out that before one can determine if the correlation dimension is any more meaningful than spectral measures it must be determined for large amounts of data from normal controls and defined patient population.

Using an argument based on a noise-corrupted sine wave Rapp et al. (1987) decided to measure 50 points per cycle for 80 cycles, giving 4000 data points. As the human alpha rhythm is approximately 10 Hz, this gives a sample interval of 2 ms. Figure 4.5.17 gives the plots for $\log C_m(r)$ versus $\log r$ for embedding dimensions 15 to 20, as well as the slope of these curves versus $\log C_m$. It is clear from the latter figure that there is a plateau region corresponding to the dimension value 2.4 ± 0.2. The sensitivity of the dimension to the number of data points used in the calculation was tested. Calculations using the third one thousand data points gave the same value of the dimension, however the degree of dispersion in the plateau is substantially decreased with the addition of more data. Rapp et al. stress that a systematic investigation is required to determine the data needed for the reliable calculations of EEG dimensions. Also, as noted earlier, the non-stationarity of the EEG time series in a given individual over time should be determined.

Rapp et al. (1987) have conducted a pilot study to determine the effect of cognitive activity on the alpha wave measured at electrode site O_2. The subject counted backwards from 300 in steps of 7. The number 7 was chosen in order that the subject could not perform the operation in a rote fashion. This pilot study is the first one designed to compare the fractal dimension in the rest state of the brain to that in the state of cognitive activity.

The pilot study yields the data depicted in Figure 4.5.13 in a slope versus $\log C_m(r)$ plot. The degree of dispersion around the plateau is greatly increased above that of the control and a dimension of 3.0 ± 0.2 is obtained, to be compared with 2.4 ± 0.2 from Figure 4.5.17. A secondary plateau is also suggested in Figure 4.5.18, this one corresponds to the higher dimension of 3.8. However, the authors note that the data does not permit a clear resolution of this object. In Figure 4.5.19 we put the results of the control and pilot study on the same slope versus $\log C_m$ graph (results provided by P. Rapp). The dimensionality of the EEG record for the individual engaged in the counting task is clearly greater than that of the control for all values of the correlation integral.

In Figure 4.5.20 the the Poincaré maps from both the control and pilot study are depicted and a remarkable difference is observed. The initiation of mental workload disrupts the structure of the resting Poincaré map, the tightly correlated points in the swirls of A and B are apparently randomized in C and D. Such an effect would, of course, be observed in such a low-dimensional projection of an attractor if the dimension of the attractor were increased.

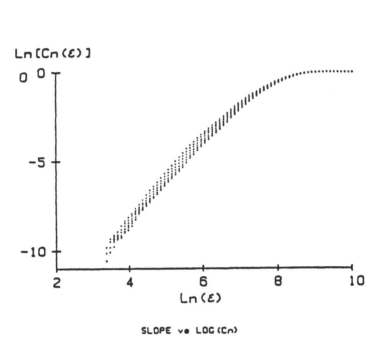

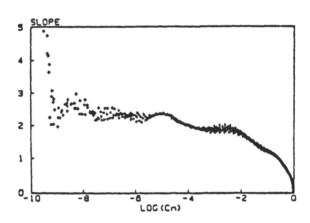

Figure 4.5.17.   Dimension calculation of the data for embedding dimensions 15 to 20. The values of C_m ran from 2 to 10 in steps of 1 and a 5-point slope calculation was used to determine v. The value of the dimension is estimated to be $2.4 \pm .2$ (from Rapp et al., 1987 with permission).

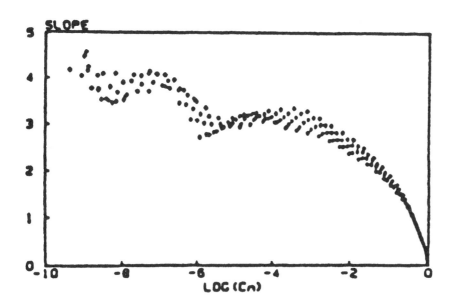

Figure 4.5.18.   Calculation of the dimension using the first 1500 data points of the signal for embedding dimension 15 to 20. The value of r ran from 2 to 10
in steps of .1. The estimated value of the dimension is 3.0±.3 (from
Rapp et al., 1987 with permission).

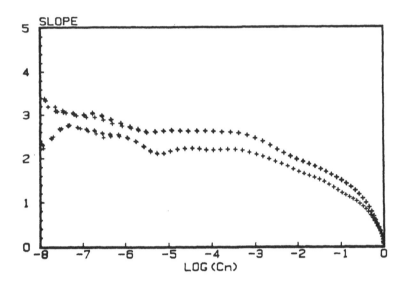

Figure 4.5.19. Slope, $d \ln C_m(r)/d \ln(r)$ versus $lnC_m(r)$ generated by two electroencephalographic time series. The lower curve corresponds to an EEG
recording at site O_z obtained from a normal, adult subject. The signal
was digitized at 500 Hz. A total of ten thousand data points were used.
During the recording, the subject was resting comfortably and his eyes
were closed. The upper curve corresponds to ten thousand points
recorded from the same subject at the same site and at the same frequency. In this latter case, the subject performed mental arithmetic during the recording. In both computations the calculations of the correlation integral was preceded by a singular value decomposition (from P.
Rapp, 1988, private communication).

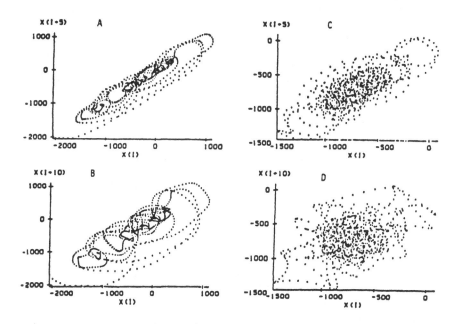

Figure 4.5.20.　Delay maps plotting the points $[X(\hat{j}), X(\hat{j}+Delay)]$. (A) The first 1000 points of the signal for eyes closed, resting. (B) The same signal as A with Delay=10. (C) The first 1000 points of the signal in Figure 4.5.19 (eyes closed, mental arithmetic) Delay = 5. (D). The same signal as in C with Delay = 10 (from Rapp et al., 1987, private communication).

References

K. Aihara, G. Matsumoto and Y. Ikegaza, "Periodic and non-periodic responses of a periodically forced Hodgkin-Huxley oscillator," J. Theor. Biol. **109**, 249-269 (1984).

S. Akselrod, D. Gordon, F. A. Ubel, P. C. Shannon, A. L. Barger and R. J. Cohen, "Power spectrum analysis for heart rate fluctuation: a quantitative probe to beat cardiovascular control," Science **213**, 220-222 (1981).

R. M. Anderson, "Directly transmitted viral and bacterial infections of man," in *The Population Dynamics of Infectious Diseases: Theory and Applications* (ed. R. M. Anderson), pp. 1-37, London, Chapman and Hall (1982).

R. M. Anderson, B. T. Grenfell and R. M. May, "Oscillator fluctuations in the incidence of infections disease and the impact of vaccination: time series analysis," J. Hyg. Camb. **93**, 587-608 (1984).

R. M. Anderson and R. M. May, Science **215**, 1053 (1982).

F. T. Angelakos and G. M. Shephard, Circ. Res. **5**, 657 (1957).

A. Arneodo, F. Argoul, P. Richetti and J. C. Roux, "The Belousov-Zhabotinskii reaction: a paradigm for theoretical studies of dynamical systems," preprint.

V.I. Arnold and A. Avez, *Ergodic Problems in Classical Mechanics*, Benjamin, New York (1968).

J. L. Aron and I. B. Schwartz, "Vaccination against rubella and measles: quantitative investigations of different policies," J. Theor. Biol. **110**, 665-679 (1984).

J. L. Aron and I.B. Schwartz, "Seasonality and period doubling bifurcations in an epidemic model," J. Theor. Biol. **110**, 665 (1984).

J. L. Aron, "Simple versus complex epidemiological models," to appear in *Applied Mathematical Ecology*, Springer-Verlag, New York, (in press).

I. Asimov, *The Human Brain*, Signet Science Lib., New York (1963).

A. Babloyantz, "Evidence of chaotic dynamics of brain activity during the sleep cycle," in *Dimensions and Entropies in Chaotic Systems*, ed. G. Mayer-Kress, Springer-Verlag, Berlin (1986).

A. Babloyantz and A. Destexhe, "Low dimensional chaos in an instance of epilepsy," Proc. Nat. Acad. Sci. USA **83**, 3515-3517 (1986).

A. Babloyantz and A. Destexhe, "Chaos in neural networks," in Proceed. Int. Conf. on Neural Networks, San Diego, June (1987).

A. Babloyantz and A. Destexhe, "Is the normal heart a periodic oscillator?" Biol. Cybern. **58**, 203-211 (1988).

A. Babloyantz, J. M. Salazar and C. Nicolis, "Evidence of chaotic dynamics during the sleep cycle," Phys. Lett. **111A**, 152-156 (1985).

M. S. Bartlett, *Stochastic Population Models in Ecology and Epidemiology*, London, Methuen (1960).

E. Basar, *Biophysical and Physiological Systems Analysis*, Addison-Wesley, London (1976).

E. Basar, H. Flohr, H. Haken and A. J. Mandell, eds. *Synergetics of the brain*, Springer-Verlag, Berlin (1983).

E. Basar, "EEG and synergetics of neural populations," in Basar et al., (1983).

E. Basar, A. Gönder, C. Ozesmi and P. Ungan, "Dynamics of brain rhythmic and evoked potentials. III Studies in the auditory pathway, recticular formation, and hippocampus during sleep," Biol. Cybernetics **20**, 161-169 (1975).

G. Benettin, L. Golgani and J. M. Strelcyn, "Kolmogorov entropy and numerical experiments," Phys. Rev. **14A**, 2338 (1976).

M. Berry, "Diffractals," J. Phys. A **12**, 781-797 (1979).

M. V. Berry and Z. V. Lewis, "On the Weierstrass-Mandelbrot fractal function," Proc. Roy. Soc. Lond. **370A**, 459 (1980).

T. H. Bullock, R. Orkand and A. Grinnel, *Introduction to the Nervous Systems*, W.H. Freeman, San Francisco (1981).

H. T. Chang, "The evoked potentials," in *Handbook of Physiology, Vol. I*, pp 299-314, J. Field, ed., Am. Physical Society, Wash. D.C. (1959).

D. L. Cohn, "Optimal systems. Parts I and II," Bull. Math. Biophys. **16**, 59-74 (1955); **17**, 219-227 (1954).

P. Collet and J. P. Eckmann, *Iterated Maps on the Interval as Dynamical Systems*, Birkhäuser, Bassel (1980).

M. Conrad, "What is the use of chaos?" in *Chaos*, ed. A.V. Holden, Manchester University Press, Manchester UK (1986).

J. P. Crutchfield, D. Donnelly, D. Farmer, G. Jones, N. Packard and R. Shaw, Phys. Lett. **76**, 1 (1980).

J. P. Crutchfield, J. D. Farmer, N. H. Packard and R. S. Shaw, "Chaos," Scientific American, 46-57 (1987).

J. H. Curry, "On the Henón transformation," Commun. Math. Phys. **68**, 129 (1979).

L. Danziger and G. L. Elmergreen, "Mathematical theory of periodic relapsing cataonia," Bull. Math. Biophys. **16**, 15-21 (1954).

C. Darwin, *The Origin of the Species by Means of Natural Selection on the Preservation of Favored Races in the Struggle of Life* (1859).

R. Dawkins, *The Selfish Gene*, Oxford University Press, New York (1976).

K. Dietz, Lect. Notes in Biomath. **11**, 1 (1976).

E. Donchin, "Brain electrical correlates of pattern recognition," in *Signal Analysis and pattern recognition in biomedical engineering*, ed. G. F. Inbar, Wiley, New York (1975).

E. Donchin, W. Ritter and W. C. McCallum, "Dognitive psychophysiology: the endongenous components of the ERP," in *Event-related brain potentials in man*, E. Callaway, P. Tueting and S. H. Koslow eds., Academic Press, New York (1978).

F. Dyson, *Origins of Life*, Cambridge University Press, Cambridge (1985).

J. P. Eckmann, "Roads to turbulence in dissipative dynamic systems," Rev. Mod. Phys. **53**, 643 (1981).

J. P. Eckmann and D. Ruelle, "Ergodic theory of chaos and strange attractors," Rev. Mod. Phys. **57**, 617-656 (1985).

I. Ekeland, *Mathematics and the Unexpected*, The Univ. Chicago Press, Chicago (1988).

D. K. Faddeev, in *Mathematics Vol. 3*, eds. A.D. Aleksandrov, A.N. Kolmogorov and M. A. Lavrentév, MIT Press, Cambridge (1964).

D. Farmer, J. Crutchfield, H. Froehling, N. Packard and R. Shaw, "Power spectra and mixing properties of strange attractors," Ann. N. Y. Acad. Sci. **357**, 453-472 (1980).

J. D. Farmer, E. Ott and J.A. Yorke, "The dimension of Chaotic Attractors," Physica 7D, 153-180 (1983).

J. Feder, *Fractals*, Plenum Press, New York (1988).

M. J. Feigenbaum, "Quantitative universality for a class of nonlinear transformations," J. Stat. Phys. **19**, 25 (1978); "The universal metric properties of nonlinear transformations," J. Stat. Phys. **21**, 669 (1979).

S. D. Feit, "Characteristic exponents and strange attractors," Commun. Math. Phys. **61**, 249 (1978).

R. J. Field, "Chemical organization in time and space," Am. Sci **73**, 142-150 (1987).

J. Ford, "Directions in Classical Chaos," in *Directions in Chaos*, ed. H. Bai-Liu, World Sci., Singapore (1987).

K. Fraedrich, "Estimating the Dimension of Weather and Climate Attractors," J. Atmos. Sci. **43**, 419-432 (1986).

W. J. Freeman, *Mass action in the nervous system*, Chapter 7, Academic Press, New York, pp 489 (1975).

W. J. Freeman, "Petit mal seizures in olfactory bulb and cortex caused by runaway inhibition after exhaustion of excitation," Brain Res. Rev. **11**, 259-284 (1986).

W. J. Freeman, "Simulation of chaotic EEG patterns with a dynamic model of the olfactory system," Biol. Cybern. **56**, 139-150 (1987).

S. Freud and Breuer, *Studies in Hysteria*, (1859).

A. Fuchs, R. Friedrich, H. Haken and D. Lehmann, "Spatio-temporal analysis of multi-channel alpha EEG way series," (preprint) (1986).

R. Gjessing, "Beitrage zur Kenntnis der Pathophysiologie les katatonen stupors: I. Mitteilung uber periodische regidevierenden ketonen stupor, mit kritischen Begeun und Abschlerss." Arch Psychiat. Nervenkrankh. **96**, 391-392 (1932).

P. Glansdorf and I. Prigogine, *Thermodynamic theory of Structure, Stability and Fluctuation*, Wiley, New York (1971).

L. Glass, M. R. Guevara and R. Perez, "Bifurcation and chaos in a periodically stimulated cardiac oscillator," Physica 7D, 39-101 (1983).

A. L. Goldberger and B. J. West, "Chaos in physiology: health or disease?" in *Chaos in Biological Systems* pp 1-5, eds. A. Holton and L.F. Olsen, Plenum (1987a).

A. L. Goldberger and B. J. West, "Applications of nonlinear dynamics to clinical cardiology," in *Perspectives in biological dynamics and Theoretical Medicine*, Ann. N. Y. Acad. Sci. **504**, 195-215 (1987b).

A. L. Goldberger and B. J. West, "Fractals; a contemporary mathematical concept with a applications to physiology and medicine," Yale J. Biol. Med. **60**, 104-119 (1987c).

A. L. Goldberger, B. J. West and V. Bhargava, "Nonlinear mechanisms in physiology and pathophysiology. Toward a dynamical theory of health and disease." Proceeding of the 11th IMACS World Congress, Oslo, Norway, Vol. 2, eds. B. Wahlstrom, R. Henrikson and N. P. Sunby, North-Holland, Amsterdam (1985a).

A. L. Goldberger, L. J. Findley, M. R. Blackburn and A. J. Mandell, "Nonlinear dynamics in heart failure: Implications of long-wavelength cardiopulmonary oscillations." Am. Heart J. **107**, 612-615 (1984).

A. L. Goldberger, K. Kobalten and V. Bhargava, IEEE Trans. Biomed. Eng. **33**, 874 (1986).

A. L. Goldberger, V. Bhargava, B. J. West and A. J. Mandell, "Some observations on the question is ventricular fibrillation chaos?" Physica **19D**, 282-289 (1986).

A. L. Goldberger, V. Bhargava, B. J. West and A. J. Mandell, "On a mechanism of cardiac electrical stability: the fractal hypothesis," Biophys. J. **48**, 525-528 (1985b).

J. P. Gollub, T. O. Brunner and D. G. Danby, "Periodicity and Chaos in Coupled Nonlinear Oscillators," Science **200**, 48-50 (1978).

J. P. Gollub, E. J. Romer and J. G. Socolar, "Trajectory Divergence for Coupled Relaxation Oscillators: Measurements and Model," J. Stat. Phys. **23**, 321-333 (1980).

P. Grassberger and I. Procaccia, "Measuring the strangeness of strange attractors," Physica **9D**, 189-208 (1983a).

P. Grassberger and I. Procaccia, "Characterization of strange attractors" Phys. Rev. Lett. **50**, 346 (1983b).

P. Grassberger and I. Procaccia, "Estimation of the Kolmogorov Entropy from a Chaotic Signal," Phys. Rev.**28A**, 2591 (1983c).

H. S. Greenside, G. Ahlers, P. C. Hohenberg and R. W. Walden, "A simple stochastic model for the generation of turbulence in Rayleigh Benard convection," Physica **5D**, 322-334 (1982).

M. R. Guevara and L. Glass "Phase locking, period doubling bifurcations and chaos in a mathematical model of a periodically driven oscillator," J. Math Biol. **14** 1-23 (1982).

J. Hanley, "Electroencephlography in Psychiatric Disorders: Parts I and II," in *Directions in Psychiatry*, vol **4**, lesson 7, pp. 1-8; lesson 8, pp. 1-8 (1984).

H. Hayashi, M. Nakao and K. Hirakawa, "Chaos in the self-sustained oscillation of an excitable biological membrane under sinusoidal stimulation," Phys. Lett. **88A**, 265-268 (1982).

H. Hayashi, M. Nakao and K. Hirakawa, "Entrained, harmonic, quasiperiodic and chaotic responses of the self-sustained oscillation of *Nitella* to sinusoidal stimulation," J. Phys. Soc. Japan **52**, 344-351 (1983).

H. Hayashi, S. Ishizuka and Hirakawa, "Transition to chaos via intermittency in the Onchidium Pacemaker Neuron," Phys. Lett. **98A**, 474-476 (1983).

H. Hayashi, S. Ishizuka, M. Ohta and K. Hirakawa, "Chaotic behavior in the *Onchidium* giant neuron under sinusoidal stimulation," Phys. Lett. **88A**, 435-438 (1982).

M. Henon, "A two-dimensional mapping with a strange attractor," Comm. Math. Phys. **50**, 69 (1976).

B. Hess, Trends in Biochem, Sci. **2**, 193-195 (1977).

B. Hess and M. Markus, "Order and chaos in biochemistry," Trends in Biochem. Sci. **12**, 45-48 (1987).

J. L. Hudson and J. C. Mankin, "Chaos in the Belousov-Zhabotinsky reaction," J. Chem. Phys. **74**, 6171-6177 (1981).

B.D. Hughes, M.F. Shlesinger and E.W. Montroll, "Random walks with self-similar clusters," Proc. Natl. Acad. Sci. USA **78**, 3287-3291 (1981).

R. E. Ideker, G. J. Klein and L. Harrison Circ. Res. **63**, 1371 (1981).

N. Ikeda, "Model of bidirectional interaction between myocardial pacemakers based on the phase response curve," Biol. Cybern. **43**, 157-167 (1982).

N. Ikeda, H. Tsuruta and T. Sato, "Difference equation model of the entrainment of myocardial pacemaker cells based on the phase response wave," Biol. Cybern. **42**, 117-128 (1981).

J. B. Isreal, C. D. Wickens, G. L. Chesney and E. Donchin, "The event-related brain potential as an index of display-monitoring workload," Human Factors **22**, 211-224 (1980a).

J. B. Isreal, G. L. Chesney, C. D. Wickens and E. Donchin, "P300 and tracking difficulty: evidence for multiple resources in dual-task performance," Psychophysiology **17**, 259-273 (1980b).

T. M. Itil, "Qualitative and quantitative EEG findings in schizophrenia," Schizophrenia Bulletin **3**, 61-79 (1977).

M. E. Josephson and S. F. Seides, *Clinical Cardiac Electrophysiology: Techniques and Interpretations*, Lea and Febiger, Phil. (1979).

P. E. B. Jourdain, Introduction to *Contributions to Transfinite Numbers* (1915), by G. Cantor. Dover (1955).

E.R. Kandel, "Small Systems of Neurons," *Mind and Behavior*, R.L. Atkinson and R.C. Atkinson eds. W.H. Freeman and Co., San Francisco (1979).

C. R. Katholi, F. Urthaler, J. Macy Jr. and T. N. James, Comp. Biomed. Res. **10**, 529 (1977).

J. P. Keener, "Chaotic cardiac dynamics," in *Lectures in Applied Mathematics* **19**, 299-325 (1981).

J. Kemeny and J. L. Snell, *Mathematical Models in the Social Sciences*, MIT Press, Cambridge, Mass. (1972).

M. Kobayashi and T. Musha, IEEE Trans. on Biomedical Eng. **29**, 456-457 (1982).

G. Kolata, "Order out of chaos in computers," Science **223**, 917-919 (1984).

S. H. Koslow, A. J. Mandell and M. F. Shlesinger, eds. *Perspectives in Biological Dynamics and Theoretical Medicine*, Ann. N. Y. Acad. Sci. **504** (1987).

A. F. Kramer, E. J. Sirevaag and R. Braune, "A psychophysiological assessment of operator workload during simulated flight mission," Human Factors **29**, 145-160 (1987).

A. F. Kramer, C. D. Wickens and E. Donchin, " An analysis of the processing requirements of a complex perceptual-motor task," Human Factors **25**, 597-621 (1983).

P. Y. Ktonas, "Automated analysis of abnormal electroencephalogram," CRC Critical Reviews of Biomedical Eng. **9**, 39-97 (1983).

O. E. Lanford, in *Statistical Mechanics and Dynamical Systems*, Math. Dept. Duke Univ., Durham, N. C., Chap. 4 (1976).

M. A. Lavrentév and S. M. Nikol'skii, in *Mathematics Vol. 1*, eds. A. D. Aleksandrov, A. N. Kolmogorov and M. A. Lavrentév, MIT Press, Cambridge (1964).

S. P. Layne, G. Mayer-Kress and J. Holzfuss, "Problems associated with dimensional analysis of electroencephalogram data," in *Dimensions and Entropies in Chaotic Systems* ed. G. Mayer-Kress, Springer-Verlag, Berlin pp. 246-256, (1986).

T. Y. Li and J. A. Yorke, "Period three implies chaos," Am. Math. Mon. **82**, 985 (1975).

W. P. London and J. A. Yorke, Am. J. Epidem **98**, 453 (1973).

E. N. Lorenz, "Deterministic Nonperiodic flow," J. Atmos. Sci. **20**, 130 (1963).

A. J. Lotka, *Elements of Mathematical Biology*, Williams and Wilkins (1925): Dover (1956).

G. G. Luce, *Biological Rhythms in Human and Animal Physiology*, Dover, New York (1971).

N. MacDonald, *Trees and Networks in Biological Models*, Wiley-Interscience, Chichester (1983).

M. C. Mackey and L. Glass, "Oscillations and chaos in physiological control systems," Science **197**, 287-289 (1977).

M. C. Mackey and J. C. Milton, "Dynamical Diseases," in *Perpectives in Biological Dynamics and Theoretical Medicine*, Ann. N. Y. Acad. Sci. **504**, 16-32 (1987).

B. B. Mandelbrot, "Fractal aspects of the iteration of $z \to \lambda z (1-z)$ for complex λ and z," Ann. N. Y. Acad. Sci **357**, 249-259 (1980).

B. B. Mandelbrot, *Fractals, Form and Chance*, W. H. Freeman (1977).

B. B. Mandelbrot, *The Fractal Geometry of Nature*, W. H. Freeman (1982).

A. J. Mandell, P. V. Russo, and S. Knapp, "Strange stability in hierarchically coupled neurophysiological systems," in *Evolution of Order and Chaos in Physics, Chemistry and Biology*, ed. H. Haken, Springer-Verlag (1982).

M. Markus, D. Kuschmitz and B. Hess, "Properties of Strange Attractors in Yeast Glycoysis," Biophys. Chem. **22**, 95-105 (1985).

R. T. Malthus, *Population: The First Essay* (1798), Univ. Mich. Press, Ann Arbor (1959).

G. Matsumoto, K. Aihara, M. Ichikawa and A. Tasaki, "Periodic and nonperiodic response of membrane potentials in squid giant axons during sinusoidal current stimulation," J. Theor. Neurobiol. **3**, 1-14 (1984).

R.D. Mauldin and S.C. Williams, "On the Hausdorff dimension of some graphs," Trans. Am. Math. Soc. **298**, 793-803 (1986).

R. M. May, "Simple mathematical models with very complicated dynamics," Nature **261**, 459-467 (1976).

G. Mayer-Kress, F. E. Yates, L. Benton, M. Keidel, W. Tirsch, S. J. Pöppl and K. Geist, "Dimensional analysis of nonlinear oscillations in brain, heart and muscle," preprint (1987).

G. Mayer-Kress and S. C. Layne, "Dimensionality of the human electroencephalogram," in *Perspectives in Biological Dynamics and Theoretical Medicine* eds. S.H. Koslow, A.J. Mandell and M.F. Shlesinger, Ann. N.Y. Acad. Sci. **504**, (1987).

H. D. Modanlon and R. K. Freeman, "Sinusoidal fetal heart rate pattern: Its definition and clinical significance," Am. J. Obsts. Gynecol. **142**, 1033-1038 (1982).

G. K. Moe, W. C. Rheinboldt and J. A. Abildskov, Am. Heart J. **67**, 200 (1964).

E. W. Montroll and B. J. West, "On an enriched collection of stochastic processes," in *Fluctuation Phenomena*, 2nd ed, E. W. Montroll and J. L. Lebowitz, North-Holland Personal Library, Amsterdam (1987).

E. W. Montroll and M. F. Shlesinger, "On $1/f$ noise and distributions with long tails," PNAS **79**, 3380-3383 (1982).

F. Moss and P.V.E. McClintock, editors, *Noise in Nonlinear Dynamical Systems*, 3 volumes Cambridge University Press, Cambridge (1989).

268

T. R. Nelson and D. K. Manchester, "Morphological modeling using fractal geometries," IEEE Trans. Med. Imag. **7**, 439 (1988).

C. Nicolis and G. Nicolis, Proc. Natl. Acad. Sci. USA **83**, 536 (1986).

J. S. Nicolis and I. Tsuda, "Chaotic dynamics of information processing: The magic number seven plus minus two revisited," Bull. Math. Biol. **47**, 343-365 (1985).

J. S. Nicolis, "Chaotic dynamics applied to information processing," Rep. Prog. Phys. **49**, 1109-1196 (1986).

N. E. Nygards and J. Hulting, *Computer in Cardiology*, (IEEE Computer Society) 393 (1977).

L. F. Olsen, "An enzyme reaction with a strange attractor," Phys. Lett. **94A**, 454-457 (1983).

L. F. Olsen, and H. Degn, "Chaos in an enzyme reaction," Nature **267**, 177-178 (1977).

L. F. Olsen and H. Degn, "Chaos in biological systems," Q. Rev. Biophys. **18**, 165-225 (1985).

Y. Oono, T. Kohda, and H. Yamazaki, "Disorder parameter for chaos," J. Phys. Soc. of Japan **48**, 738-745 (1980).

A. R. Osborne and A. Provenzale, "Finite correlation dimension for stochastic systems with power law spectra," Physica **D35**, 357-381 (1989).

V. I. Oseledec, "A multiplicative ergodic theorem, Lyapunov characteristic numbers for dynamical systems," Trudy Mosk. Mat. Obsc. **19**, 179 [Moscow Math. Soc. **19**, 197 (1968)].

E. Ott, "Strange attractors and chaotic motions of dynamical systems," Rev. Mod. Phys. **57**, 655-671 (1985).

N. H. Packard, J. P. Crutchfield, J. D. Farmer and R. S. Shaw, "Geometry from a Times Series," Phys. Rev. Lett. **45**, 712-716 (1980).

S. Panchev, *Random Functions and Turbulence*, Pergamon Press, Oxford (1971).

P. J. E. Peebles, *The Large-scale Structure of the Universe*, Princeton Univ. Press (1980).

R. Pool, "Is it chaos, or is it just noise?" in Science **243**, 25 (1989).

J. C. Principe and J. R. Smith, "Microcomputer-based system for the detection and quantification of petit mal epilepsy," Comput. Biol. Med. **12**, 87-95 (1982).

P.E. Rapp, J. Exp. Biol. **81**, 281-306 (1979).

P. E. Rapp, R. A. Latta and A. I. Mees, "Parameter-dependent transitions and the optimal control of dynamic diseases," Bull. Math. Biol.

P. E. Rapp, I. D. Zimmerman, A. M. Albano, G. C. de Guzman, N. N. Greenbaum and T. R. Bashore, "Experimental studies of chaotic neural behavior: cellular activity and electroencephalogram signals," in *Nonlinear Oscillations in Biology and Chemistry* ed. H.G. Othmer, PP. 175-205, Springer-Verlag (1987).

P. E. Rapp, I. D. Zimmerman, A. M. Albano, G. C. de Guzman and N. N. Greenbaum, "Dynamics of spontaneous neural activity in the simian motor cortex: the dimension of chaotic neurons," Phys. Lett. **110A**, 335-338 (1985).

N. Rashevsky, *Mathematical Biophysics Physico - Mathematical Foundations of Biology*, vol. 2, 3rd rev. ed., Dover, New York (1960).

L.F. Richardson, "Atmospheric diffusion shown on a distance-neighbor graph," Proc. Roy. Soc. Lond. A **110**, 709 (1926).

J. Rinzel and R. N. Miller, Math Biosci. **49**, 27 (1980).

A. I. Ritzenberg, D. R. Adam and R. J. Cohen "Period multiplying evidence for nonlinear behaviour of the canine heart," Nature **307**, 157 (1984).

F. Rohrer, "Flow resistance in human air passages and the effect of irregular branching of the bronchial system on the respiratory process in various regions of the lungs." Pflugers Arch. **162**, 225-99. Repr. 1975: *Translations in Respiratory Physiology*, ed. J. B. West, Stroudsburg, PA: Dowden, Hutchinson and Ross.

O. E. Rössler, "An Equation for Continuous Chaos," Phys. Lett. **57A**, 397-398 (1976).

O. Rössler, "Continuous chaos-four prototype equations," in *Bifurcation Theory and Applications to Scientific Disciplines*, Ann. N.Y. Acad. Sci. **316**, 376-392 (1978).

J. C. Roux, J. S. Turner, W. D. McCormick and H. L. Swinney, "Experimental observations of complex dynamics in a chemical reaction," in *Nonlinear Problems: Present and Future*, eds. A. R. Bishop, D. K. Campbell and B. Nicolaenko, 409-422, North-Holland, Amsterdam (1982).

J. C. Roux, R. M. Simoyi and H. L. Swinney, "Observation of a strange attractor," Physica **D8**, 257 (1983).

W. M. Schaffer and M. Kott, "Nearly one dimensional dynamics in an epidemic," J. Theor. Biol. **112**, 403-427 (1985).

W. M. Schaffer, "Can nonlinear dynamics elucidate mechanisms in ecology and epidemiology?" IMAJ Math Appl. Med. Biol. **2**, 221-252 (1985).

K. Schmidt-Nielson, *Scaling, Why is Animal Size so Important?*, Cambridge University Press, Cambridge, London (1984).

I. B. Schwartz, "Multiple stable recurrent outbreaks and predictability in seasonally forced nonlinear epidemic models," J. Math. Biol. **21**, 347 (1985).

I. B. Schwartz and H. L. Smith, "Infinite subharmonic bifurcations in an SEIR model," J. Math. Biol. **18**, 233-253 (1983).

L. A. Segal, *Modeling Dynamic Phenomena in Molecular and Cellular Biology*, Cambridge Univ. Press, London (1984).

M. Sernetz, B. Gelléri and J. Hoffman, "The organism as bioreactor. Interpolation of the reduction law of metabolism in terms of heterogeneous catalysis and fractal structure." J. Theor. Biol. **117**, 209-230 (1985).

R. Shaw, "Strange attractors, chaotic behavior, and information flow," Z. Naturforsch **36A**, 80-112 (1981).

R. Shaw, *The Dripping Faucet as a Model Chaotic System*, Ariel Press, Santa Cruz, CA (1984).

A. Siegel, C. L. Grady and A. F. Mirsky, "Prediction of spike-wave bursts in disence epilepsy by EEG power-spectra signals," Epilepsia. **23**, 47-60 (1982).

D. Sigeti and W. Horsthemke, "High frequency spectra for systems subject to noise," Phys. Rev. **A35**, 2276-2282 (1987).

R. H. Simoyi, A. Wolf and H. L. Swinney, "One-dimensional dynamics in a multicomponent chemical reaction," Phys. Rev. Lett. **49**, 245-248 (1982).

J. M. Smith and R. J. Cohen, Proc. Natl. Acad. Sci. **81**, 233 (1984).

F. Takens, in *Lecture Notes in Mathematics, 898*, ed. D. A. Rand and L. S. Young, Springer-Verlag, Berlin (1981).

G. R. Taylor, *The Great Evolution Mystery*, Harper and Row (1983).

D. W. Thompson, *On Growth and Form*, 2nd Ed., Cambridge Univ. Press (1963), original (1917).

E.E. Underwood and K. Banerji, "Fractals in fractography," Mat. Sci. and Eng. **80**, 1-14 (1986).

B. van der Pol and J. van der Mark, Extr. arch. neerl. physiol. de l'homme et des animaux **14**, 418 (1929).

B. van der Pol and J. van der Mark, "The heartbeat considered as a relaxation oscillator and an electrical model of the heart," Phil. Mag. **6**, 763 (1928).

D. M. Vassalle, Circ. Res. **41**, 269 (1977).

P. F. Verhulst, Mem. Acad. Roy. Bruxelles **28**, 1 (1844).

M.V. Volkenshstein, *Biophysics*, MIR pub., Moscow (1983).

R.F. Voss, "Fractals in nature: from characterization to simulation," in *The Science of Fractal Images*, eds. H. Peitgen and D. Saupe, Springer-Verlag, New York (1988).

J. L. Waddington, M. J. MacColloch and J. E. Sambrooks, Experientia, **35**, 1197 (1979).

R. C. Watt and S. R. Hameroff, "Phase space reconstruction and dimensional analysis of EEG," in *Perspectives in Biological Dynamics and Theoretical Medicine*, eds. S. H. Koslow, A. J. Mandell and M. F. Shlesinger, N. Y. Acad. Sci. **504**, (1987).

B. J. West, *An Essay on the Importance of Being Nonlinear*, Lect. Notes in Biomathematics **62**, Springer-Verlag, Berlin (1985).

B. J. West, "Fractals, Intermittency and Morphogenesis," in *Chaos in Biological Systems*, pp. 305-317, eds. A. Holton and L. F. Olsen, Plenum (1987).

B. J. West, "Fractals in Physiology," in *Dynamic Patterns in Complex Systems*, eds. J. A. S. Kelso, A. J. Mandell and M. F. Shlesinger, World Science, Singapore (1988).

B. J. West and A. L. Goldberger, "Physiology in fractal dimensions," Am. Sci. **75**, 354-365 (1987).

B. J. West and J. Salk, "Complexity, Organization and Uncertainty," E. J. Oper. Res. **30**, 117-128 (1987).

B. J. West, A. L. Goldberger, G. Rovner and V. Bhargava, "Nonlinear dynamics of the heartbeat I. The AV junction: Passive conduit or active oscillator?" Physica **17D**, 198-206 (1985).

B. J. West, V. Bhargava and A. L. Goldberger, "Beyond the principle of similitude: renormalization in the bronchial tree," J. Appl. Physiol. **60**, 189-197 (1986).

H. Whitney, Ann. Math. **37**, 645 (1936).

C. D. Wickens, "Human workload measurement," in *Mental Workload; Its theory and measurement*, N. Moray ed., Plenum, New York (1979).

C. D. Wickens, J. B. Isreal and E. Donchin, "The event related potential as an index of task workload," in *Proceeding of the human factors Society 21st Annual meeting*, eds. A. S. Neal and R. F. Palasek, San Francisco October (1977).

C. Wickens, A. Kramer, L. Vanasse and E. Donchin, "Performance of concurrent tasks: a psychophysiological analysis of the reciprocity of information-processing resources," Science **221**, 1080-1082 (1983).

E. R. Wiebel, *Morphometry of the Human Lung*, Academic Press, New York (1963).

E. R. Wiebel and D. M. Gomez, "Architecture of the human lung," Science **137**, 577-585 (1962).

N. Wiener, *Time Series*, MIT press, Cambridge, Mass. (1949).

N. Wiener, *Cybernetics*, MIT Press, Cambridge, Mass. (1963).

N. Wiener, *Harmonic Analysis*, MIT Press, Cambridge Mass (1964).

K. G. Wilson, "Problems in physics with many scales of length," Sci. Am. **241**, 158-179 (1979).

T. A. Wilson, "Design of the bronchial tree," Nature Lond. **18**, 668-669 (1967).

A. T. Winfree, J. Thor. Biol. **16**, 15 (1977).

A. T. Winfree, J. Thor. Biol. **249**, 144 (1984).

A. Wolf, J. B. Swift, H. L. Swinney and J. A. Vastano, "Determining Lyapunov exponents from a time series," Physica **16D**, 285-317 (1985).

S. J. Worley, J. L. Swain and P. G. Colavita, Am. J. Cariol. **5**, 813 (1985).

J. A. Yorke and E. D. Yorke, "Metastable Chaos: The transition to sustained chaotic behavior in the Lorenz model," J. Stat. Phys. **21**, 263 (1979).

INDEX